THE NEW AIR FRYER COO
FOR BEGINNERS Ul_

WITH COLOUR PICTURES

Many healthy, quick, and delicious recipes for every day with tips and tricks for perfect frying.

Lauren O'Sullivan

What is an Air Fryer?

An air fryer is an appliance that typically has an egg shape with a removable basket on which the dishes to be cooked are placed. It uses the concept of cooking with air at high temperatures that reach up to 200°c, allowing a very healthy "frying-not-frying" of fresh and frozen foods. Therefore, abandon the idea of frying in dishes in a lot of oil; the amount of oil used in the air fryer is a few teaspoons or some spritz. Frying in a lot of boiling oil is as good as it is "dangerous," especially if it is "abused" or not given due attention. In the air fryer, the oil never reaches the smoke point and, therefore, is not toxic as the one used for deep frying could be.

The hot air, which reaches high temperatures, circulates in the air fryer chamber, allowing the dishes to be cooked evenly both externally and internally. In this way, you can cook meat, fish, vegetables, and a thousand other dishes in just a few minutes. In short, you can create many recipes with the air fryer. Meat cooked in an air fryer is juicy, very tender, and soft; excess fats drip to the bottom and do not remain inside the meat, giving it an exceptional flavour.

How does the air fryer work?

The air fryer is much more and in addition to its main purpose (the air cooking of food for light and healthy fried foods), it is also an appliance that acts as an oven for the gratin of many recipes (pasta dishes such as lasagne, rice, pasta), for cooking desserts and cakes of all kinds, savoury pies, muffins, focaccias, pizzas, etc.
It allows you to roast, grill, and gratin as in the oven but in much less time! It has been proven that in the best performing models, the air fryer eliminates excess fat, even up to 50%, without altering the taste of the food, however, giving the right crunchiness typical of fried foods.

Which air fryer to choose?

The power: it must be at least 1500W but if it reaches 1800W or 2000W, it's even better. In this way, the power consumption is not really very low but if you think of the same dishes that you could cook in the oven (which completely cooks in twice as long a time and which must be preheated) or on an induction hob (for cooking in a pan) or on an electric plate (for grilling meat, fish, and vegetables), you will immediately realize the savings not only in economic terms but also in time and health terms: less fat and less fried.

The capacity: there are different sizes, more than aesthetic but of capacity of the basket. Capacity bands are typically:

• up to 2 people (800g or 2.5l)
• up to 3 people (1.2kg or 3.5l)
• for 4 or more people (1.4kg or 5.5l format)

In the air fryer, you can use all the moulds that you typically use for cooking in the oven but always ensure that the quality is good and that they are suitable for cooking in the oven at high temperatures.

The dimensions: make sure of the space you have available because it is not really small; especially having the removable basket that should rest on the top. Also remember that it emits hot air, so it is preferable not to be used on delicate surfaces such as glass, plastic and so on.

What are the benefits?

• Possibility of making fried foods with less fat, lighter, and healthier.
• Possibility to consume fried foods occasionally, even for those with cholesterol problems.
• Not reaching the smoke point, the oil does not risk becoming toxic.
• Less dirt and no bad smells.
• Greater hygiene.
• Quick and easy cleaning of the machine.
• Cooking without risk of domestic accidents.
• Savings in the amount of oil used.

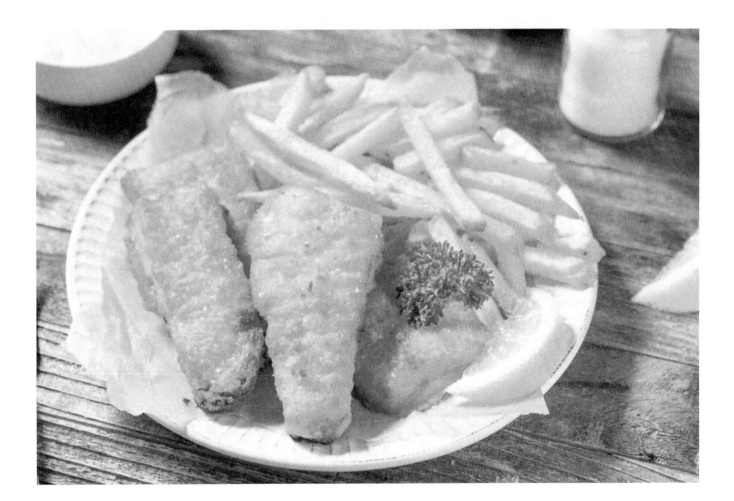

POULTRY RECIPES

CHICKEN THIGHS

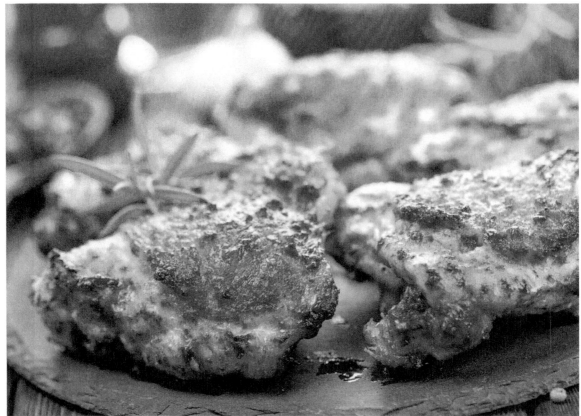

- **Preparation: 5 minutes**
- **Cooking: 12 minutes**
- **Difficulty: Very easy**
- **Servings: 2**

INGREDIENTS
- 4 Chicken thighs
- 1 teaspoon or 2-3 spritz Olive oil
- ½ teaspoon of Mixed herbs
- 1 sprig Rosemary
- Fine salt to taste

PREPARATION
Remove the skin from the chicken and place the legs in a pan. Spray them with the 2-3 spritz of olive oil or brush on the olive oil if you don't have your oil in a spray bottle.
Then, season them with fine salt, herb mixture, and rosemary.
Massage the thighs so that they completely absorb the flavours.

COOKING CHICKEN THIGS IN AIR FRYER
Put a glass of water on the bottom of the air fryer (a little more or a little less, depending on the size of your chicken thighs).

This will help prevent drops of fat from burning on the bottom and emitting smoke. Then, place the chicken thighs directly on the basket without parchment paper or moulds. Run the air fryer at 200°c and turn them after about 5 minutes. Continue cooking for another 6-7 minutes.

CHICKEN WINGS

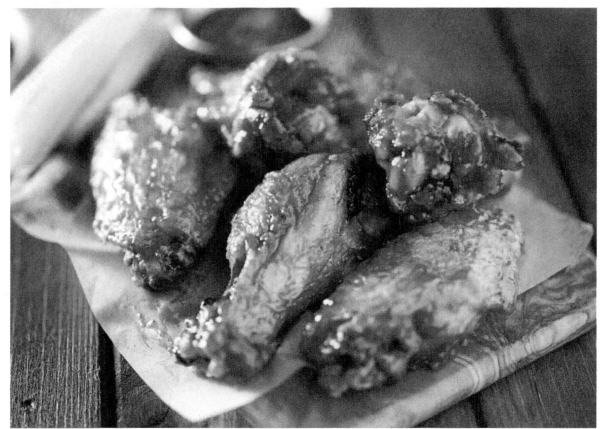

- **Preparation: 10 minutes**
- **Cooking time: 12 minutes**
- **Difficulty: Very easy**
- **Servings: 3**

INGREDIENTS
- 500g Chicken wings at room temperature
- 1 tablespoon Olive oil
- ½ tablespoon Garlic powder
- Paprika
- Salt and pepper to taste.

PREPARATION
In a bowl, add your chicken wings, then pour the tablespoon of olive oil, garlic powder, and paprika (depending on how spicy you want the dish, you might use up to ½ tablespoon). Add salt and pepper. Massage in the spices and leave the chicken wings to marinate for at least 10 minutes.

COOKING SPICY CHICKEN WINGS IN AIR FRYER
Preheat the air fryer to 180°c.
Place the chicken wings in the basket and insert into the air fryer. Set the timer to 12 minutes and all the chicken wings to cook. They will become crispy, and that's when you know they are ready. Remove the wings and serve hot with various sauces.

CHICKEN BURGER

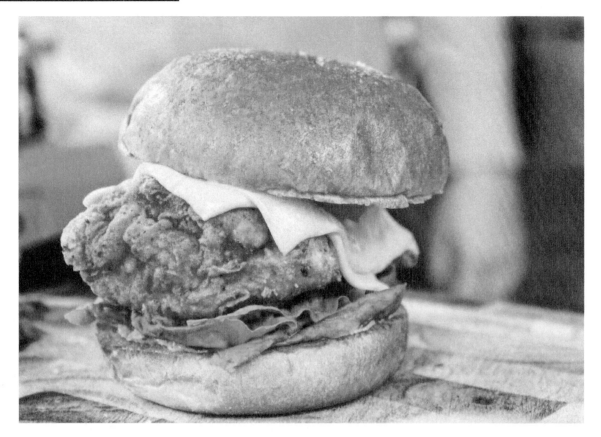

- **Preparation: 10 minutes**
- **Cooking: 7 minutes**
- **Difficulty: Very easy**
- **Servings: 2**

INGREDIENTS
- 500g Minced chicken
- 1 tablespoon Grated parmesan
- ½ tablespoon Herbs of your choice
- Fine salt to taste

PREPARATION
Work the minced chicken directly into a bowl with a spatula. Add the herbs, parmesan, and salt and mix, forming a dough. Divide the dough into 4 equal parts (you will get burgers of 125g each). Shape each block into balls.
Use the appropriate tool or a simple pastry mould with a maximum diameter of 10-12 cm. Put the ball inside the mould and press so as to perfectly distribute the dough and give the burger shape. If necessary, you can also use film.

COOKING CHICKEN BURGER IN AIR FRYER
Place your chicken patties on the basket and set the air fryer at 160°c for 3-4 minutes, then increase the temperature to 180°c and cook for another two minutes, then finish them off at 200°c.

SWEET PAPRIKA CHICKEN

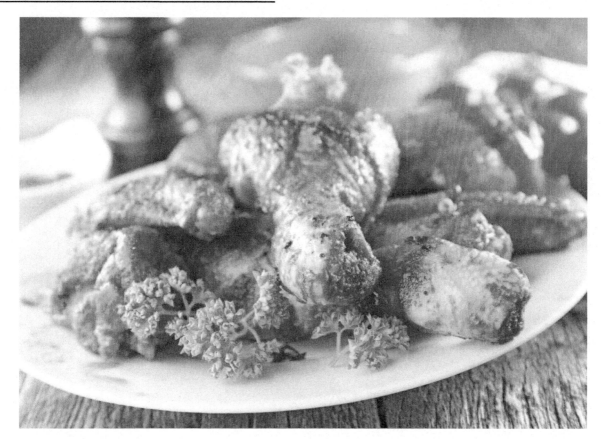

- **Preparation: 20 minutes**
- **Cooking time: 25 minutes**
- **Difficulty: Easy**
- **Servings: 3**

INGREDIENTS
- 6 Chicken legs
- 1 teaspoon Sweet paprika
- 50g Breadcrumbs
- 5g Rosemary leaves
- Salt to taste
- A little extra virgin olive oil

PREPARATION
In a small bowl, add the breadcrumbs, salt, paprika, and rosemary leaves.
Mix everything, then using a kitchen brush, brush the chicken legs with very little oil.
Dip the chicken legs in the flavoured breadcrumbs and coat evenly.

COOKING CHICKEN WITH SWEET PAPRIKA IN AIR FRYER
Preheat the air fryer using the appropriate function then place the chicken legs inside. Cook for about 15 minutes at 200°c and for 10 additional minutes at 170°c.

CRUNCHY CHICKEN BREAST NUGGETS

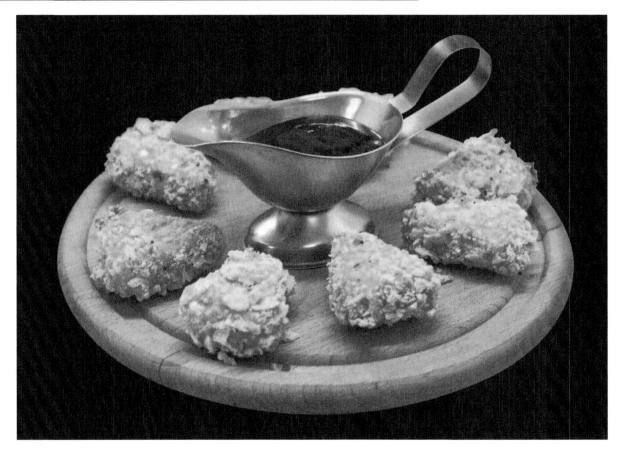

- **Preparation: 15 minutes**
- **Cooking time: 20 minutes**
- **Difficulty: Easy**
- **Servings: 2**

INGREDIENTS
- 300g Chicken breast
- 40g Rolled oats
- 1 egg
- 50g Flour
- 10g Parsley
- Salt and pepper to taste

PREPARATION
Cut the chicken breast into bite-sized pieces and set aside. Season the oat flakes with salt, pepper, and parsley (you can add other spices of your liking). Bread the breast pieces by passing them first in the flour, then in the egg, and finally in the seasoned oat flakes.

COOKING CRISPY NUGGETS IN AIR FRYER
Place the chicken nuggets in the air fryer and cook for about 20 minutes at a temperature of 200°c.

CHICKEN CUTLETS

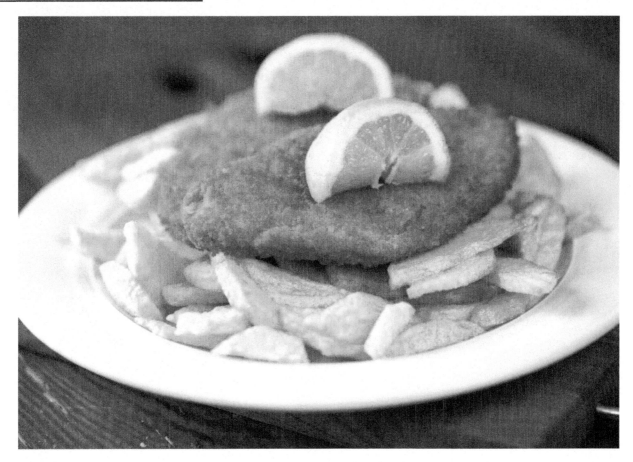

- **Preparation: 10 minutes**
- **Cooking time: 10 minutes**
- **Difficulty: Very easy**
- **Servings: 4**

INGREDIENTS
- 4 slices Chicken breast
- 80g Parmesan breading
- 30ml Olive oil
- Fine salt to taste

PREPARATION
Beat the chicken breast slices if they are very thick. You can buy it either already sliced or can slice the whole breast to the thickness you prefer. Consider that the thicker the chicken slices, the more cooking needed.
Prepare the parmesan breading without olive oil; add salt to taste. Coat chicken with olive oil. Then pass the slices of chicken breast in the breading, ensuring that it coats evenly.

COOKING CHICKEN CUTLETS IN AIR FRYER
Place the cutlets on the basket of the air fryer, without parchment paper or trays. Spritz them with olive oil on the side that is up, then cook at 200°c for 4 minutes or until they are golden. Then, turn them and spritz with olive oil again, cooking them for another 4 minutes.

YOGURT CHICKEN SKEWERS

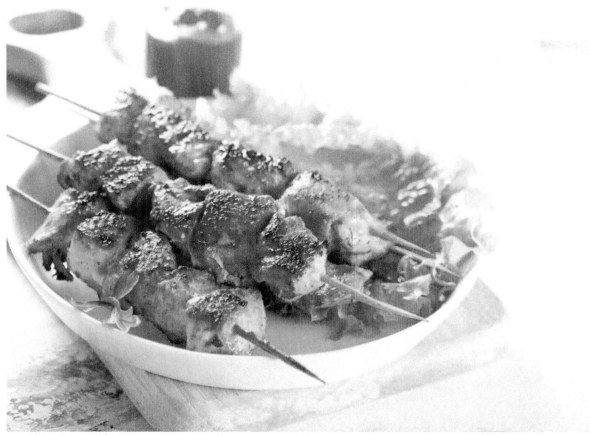

- **Preparation time: 3 hours**
- **Cooking time: 10 minutes**
- **Difficulty: Medium**
- **Servings: 3**

INGREDIENTS
- 450g Deboned chicken thighs
- 120g Greek yogurt
- 20ml of olive oil
- 2g Paprika
- 1g Ground cumin
- 1g Chopped red pepper
- Juice of 1 lemon
- Peel from 1 lemon• Salt
- 1g Ground black pepper
- 4 Cloves minced garlic
- 2 Wooden skewers

PREPARATION
Mix together the yogurt, lemon juice, lemon peel, paprika, cumin, olive oil, red pepper, salt, pepper and garlic in a large bowl.
Add the chicken to the marinade and marinate in the fridge for 2-3 hours. Cut the chicken thighs into 40mm pieces and skewer them on the skewers.

COOKING YOGURT CHICKEN SKEWERS IN AIR FRYER
Place the skewers in the preheated fryer and spray with cooking spray. Cook at 200°c for 10 minutes.

CHICKEN WINGS WITH HONEY

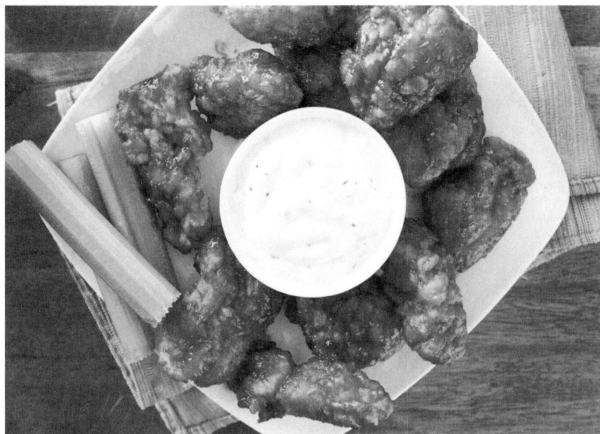

- **Preparation: 10 Minute**
- **Cooking time: 30 minutes**
- **Difficulty: Easy**
- **Servings: 3**

INGREDIENTS
- 2g Smoked paprika
- 2g Garlic powder
- 2g Onion powder
- Salt to taste
- 2g Black pepper
- 25g Corn starch
- 450g Chicken wings
- Non-stick cooking spray
- 90g Honey
- 100g Sriracha
- 15ml Rice wine vinegar
- 5ml Sesame oil

PREPARATION
Mix together the smoked paprika, garlic powder, onion powder, salt, black pepper, and corn starch.
Toss the wings in the seasoned corn starch until they are evenly covered. Whisk together honey, sriracha, rice wine vinegar, and sesame oil in a large bowl. Set this aside.

COOKING CHICKEN WINGS WITH HONEY IN AIR FRYER
Place the wings in the preheated fryer.

Set the timer to 30 minutes and place the chicken inside the basket. Shake the basket halfway through cooking. Place the cooked wings in the sauce until well covered and serve.

BARBECUE CHICKEN

- **Preparation: 30 minutes**
- **Cooking time 20 minutes**
- **Difficulty: Medium**
- **Servings: 4**

INGREDIENTS
- 3g Smoked paprika
- 5g Garlic powder
- 3g Onion powder
- 4g Chilli powder
- 7g Cane sugar
- Salt
- 2g Ground cumin
- 1g Cayenne pepper
- 1g Black pepper
- 1g White pepper
- 450g Chicken legs
- 230g Chicken wings
- Barbecue sauce

PREPARATION
Combine all the ingredients in a small bowl, except the chicken. Then add the chicken and leave to marinate for 30 minutes.

COOKING BARBECUE CHICKEN IN AIR FRYER
Turn on the air fryer and set the temperature to 200°c. Place the chicken in the preheated fryer. Set the timer to 20 minutes. Brush the chicken with a little barbecue sauce every 6-7 minutes. Remove the chicken from the fryer when it is done cooking. Serve with barbecue sauce.

ROAST CHICKEN

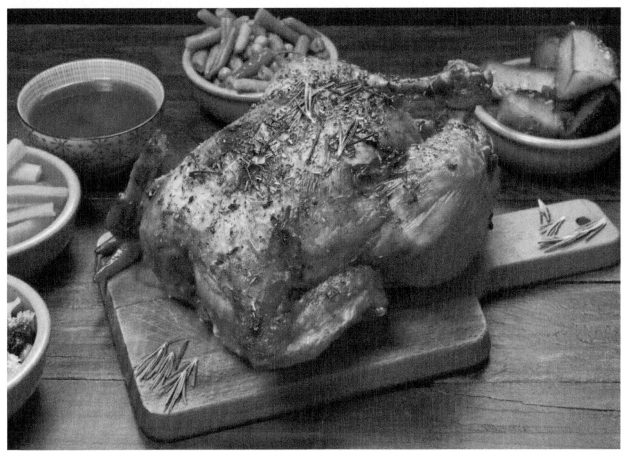

- **Preparation: 10 minutes plus time to marinate**
- **Cooking time: 40 minutes**
- **Difficulty: Very easy**
- **Servings: 4**

INGREDIENTS
- 1 Whole Chicken (about 1 kg)
- 2 Lemons
- 3 tablespoons Extra virgin olive oil
- 1 tablespoon Parsley
- 2 Cloves of garlic
- 1 tablespoon Oregano
- 2 sprigs Rosemary
- Salt to taste

PREPARATION
In a bowl, squeeze the juice of a lemon and add chopped garlic cloves, extra virgin olive oil, oregano, rosemary leaves, and salt. Beat everything with a fork to create the marinade and then put the chicken in the bowl and coat it, massaging both the outside and the inside in order to distribute the mixture well.
Add the second lemon sliced and let the chicken marinate for at least 1 hour.

COOKING ROAST CHICKEN IN AIR FRYER
Put the chicken in the fryer basket so that the juices go down during cooking and cook it for 20 minutes at 160°c, the skin will become crunchy, and the meat inside will cook gently without becoming dry and stringy. After the time has elapsed, cook for another 20 minutes at 180°c to brown the chicken well.

CHICKEN LEGS WITH LEMON

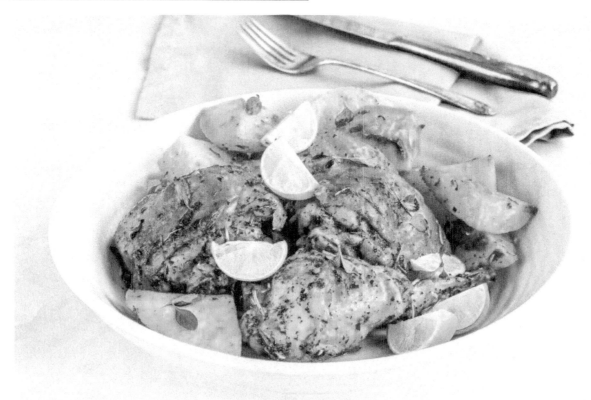

- **Preparation: 10 minutes**
- **Cooking time: 20 minutes**
- **Difficulty: Very easy**
- **Servings: 3**

INGREDIENTS
- 30ml Olive oil
- 1 Lemon
- 5g Paprika
- 5g Garlic powder
- Salt to taste
- 1g Dried oregano
- 1g Grounded black pepper
- 2g Cane sugar
- 6 Chicken legs with skin on

PREPARATION
Mix together the olive oil, juice from lemon, lemon zest, garlic powder, paprika, salt, oregano, black pepper, and cane sugar in a bowl. Add the chicken legs to the marinade and leave to rest for 30 minutes.

COOKING IN AIR FRYER
Turn on the air fryer, adjust to 195°c. Place the chicken legs in the preheated fryer.
Adjust the timer to 20 minutes and press start. Remove after 20 minutes.

CHICKEN BREAST IN SOY SAUCE

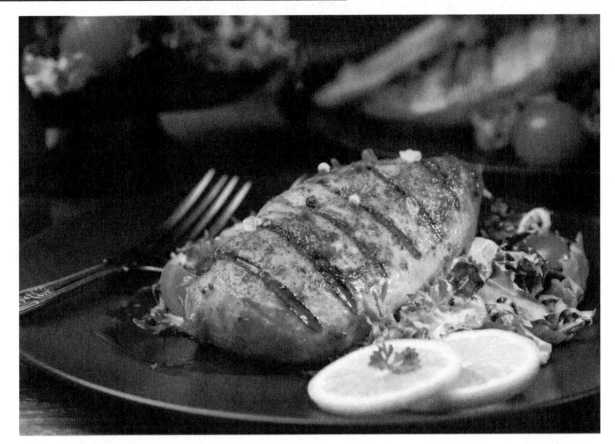

- **Preparation: 5 minutes**
- **Cooking: 8 minutes**
- **Difficulty: Easy**
- **Servings: 2**

INGREDIENTS
- 300g Chicken breast
- 15g Honey
- 1 Lime for garnish
- 25ml Soy sauce
- 3g Grated ginger
- 1g Paprika
- 1 teaspoon Oil of your choice
- Salt and pepper

PREPARATION
Remove skin from chicken breast and place in a bowl. Add the soy sauce, honey, grated ginger, paprika, salt and pepper. Oil the basket in the air fryer.

COOKING CHICKEN BREAST IN SOY SAUCE IN THE FRYER
Put the chicken breasts in the previously oiled baskets and cook at 170°c for about 8 minutes. Garnish with some lime zest and juice.

BEEF, PORK, AND LAMB RECIPES

BEEF MEATBALLS

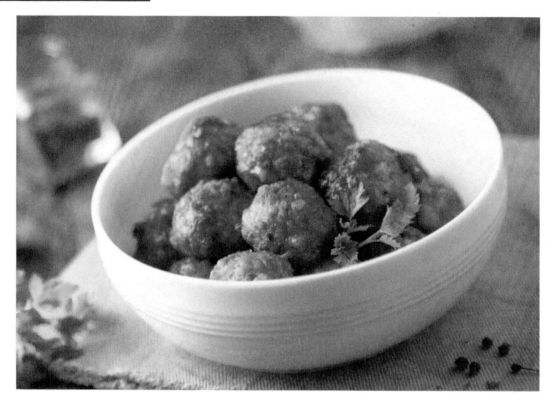

- **Preparation: 5 minutes**
- **Cooking time: 12 minutes**
- **Difficulty: Very easy**
- **Servings: 4**

INGREDIENTS
- 500g Beef
- 1 egg
- 50g Breadcrumbs
- 2g Black pepper
- Fine salt
- 80g Parmesan
- 2g Garlic powder
- 15ml Olive oil

PREPARATION
To prepare meatballs, put the minced meat into a bowl with 1 large egg, salt, pepper, parmesan, the breadcrumbs, and garlic powder (or a clove of garlic chopped). Mix all the ingredients well, so that they are well combined with the meat.
Form the meatballs; in a deep dish, add 15 ml of olive oil and roll into the meat mixture. Then portion and form into balls.

COOKING BEEF MEATBALLS IN AIR FRYER
Place the meatballs in the perforated basket of the air fryer and cook for 7 minutes at 180°c, then turn them if necessary and cook for another 5 minutes at 200°c.

BEEF STEAK

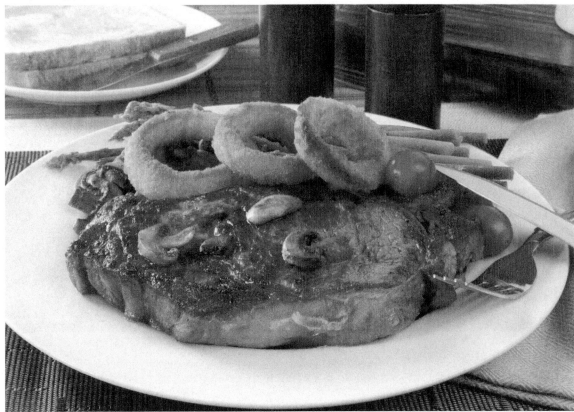

- **Preparation: 5 minutes**
- **Cooking time: 10 minutes**
- **Difficulty: Very easy**
- **Servings: 1**

INGREDIENTS
- 1 Beef steak
- Half a peeled onion
- 1 tablespoon EVO oil
- 1 teaspoon Aromatic herbs
- Salt and pepper

PREPARATION
Peel the onion and cut it into rings, put the rings in cold water for at least 5 minutes. Remove the meat from the refrigerator 30 minutes before you need to cook it in the air fryer (in this way, it will cook evenly during the cooking process).
Put the onion rings, salt, pepper, herbs, and extra virgin olive oil on the meat.

COOKING BEEF STEAK IN AIR FRYER
Turn on the fryer and set the temperature to 180°c. Put the meat in the basket of the oil-free fryer, set the cooking timer to 10 minutes.

BEEF BURGER

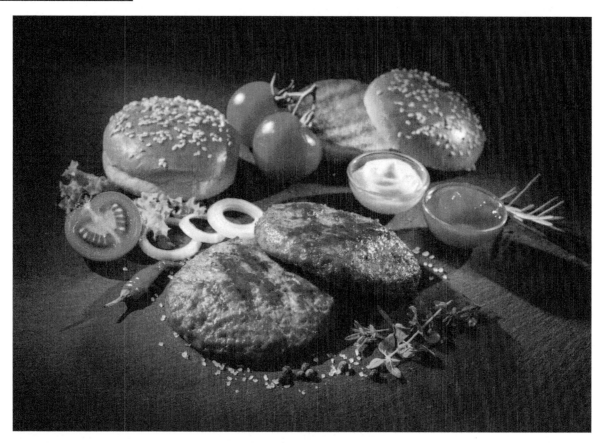

- **Preparation: 50 minutes**
- **Cooking time: 10 minutes**
- **Difficulty: Easy**
- **Servings: 4**

INGREDIENTS
- 450g Ground beef
- Salt to taste
- 1g Black pepper
- 6ml Worcestershire sauce
- 5g Dijon mustard
- 1 Small onion, grated
- 1 Beaten egg
- 1 tablespoon Olive oil
- 4 slices Cheddar cheese
- Buns for serving

PREPARATION
Mix together the ground beef, the grated onion, Dijon mustard, Worcestershire sauce, black pepper, egg and grated onion until well combined.
Form 4 beef patties and let them sit in the refrigerator for 35-40 minutes.

COOKING BEEF BURGER IN AIR FRYER
Turn on the air fryer and set the temperature to 180°c.
Brush the patties with oil and put the burgers in the preheated fryer. Set the time to 10 minutes and press start.
Flip the burgers halfway through cooking to ensure even browning. Add cheddar slices and serve.

PORK RIBS IN BBQ SAUCE

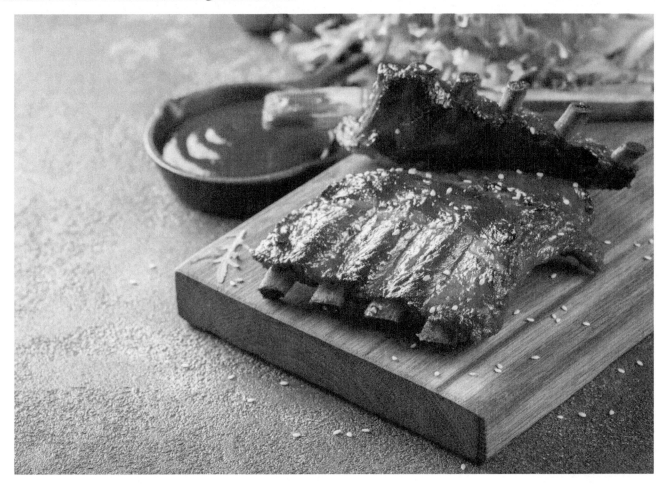

- **Preparation: 10 minutes**
- **Cooking time: 25 minutes**
- **Difficulty Very easy**
- **Servings: 2**

INGREDIENTS
- 600g Pork ribs
- Fine salt to taste
- 100ml Barbeque sauce
- 2 spritz Olive oil

PREPARATION
First of all, leave the ribs at room temperature for about 20 minutes before cooking them. Cooking it too cold tends to harden the meat and affect the cooking. Then, season it with a little salt and spray it with only 2 spritz of oil.

COOKING PORK RIBS IN BBQ SAUCE IN AIR FRYER
Pour half a glass of water into the bottom of the basket to prevent the grease from producing smoke. Place the ribs directly on the rack and operate the air fryer at 180°c. Cook for 10 minutes then brush them with the barbeque sauce and continue for another 10 minutes.
Turn them and brush them on the other side, then continue cooking at 200°c for 5 minutes.

ROAST PORK

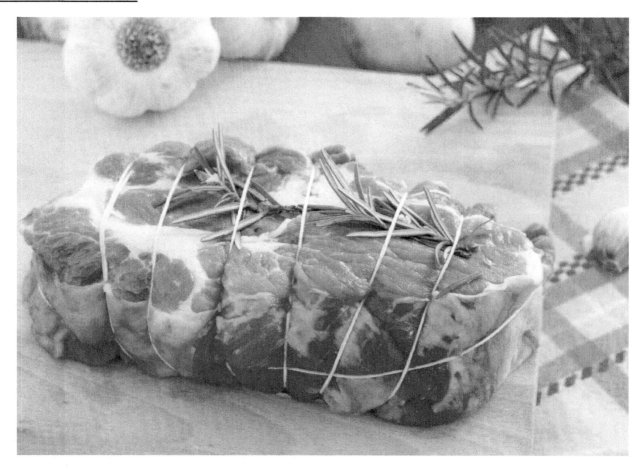

- **Preparation: 10 minutes**
- **Cooking time: 50 minutes**
- **Difficulty: Easy**
- **Servings: 4**

INGREDIENTS
- 1kg Pork loin
- Salt and pepper to taste
- 1 sprig Rosemary

PREPARATION
For this recipe, it is best to buy pork that is wrapped in a net. Otherwise, wrap your loin in a next or tie together with a length of cooking string to start with. Take the loin and season it with salt and pepper, put a nice sprig of rosemary in the net.

COOKING ROAST OF PORK IN AIR FRYER
Put it in the air fryer, start the chops program for 30 minutes at 180°c and then for another 20 minutes at 200°c. Leave to rest for 15 minutes before serving.

KOREAN STYLE BEEF SKEWERS

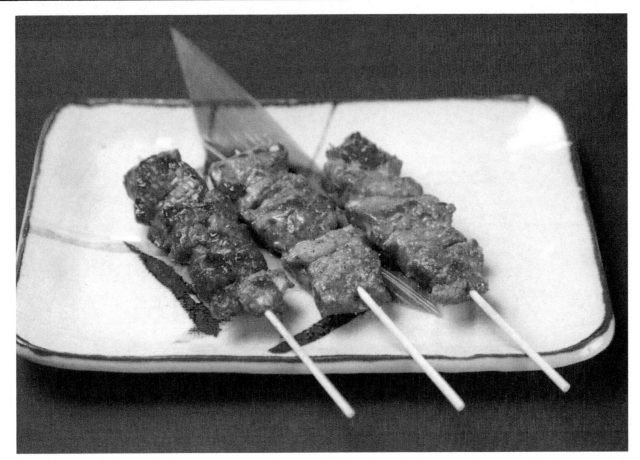

- **Preparation time: 1 hour**
- **Cooking time: 10 minutes**
- **Difficulty: Very easy**
- **Servings: 3**

INGREDIENTS
- 450g Diced beef
- 15ml Soy sauce
- 15ml Sesame oil
- 15ml Honey
- 5ml Wine vinegar
- 2 Wooden skewers
- Salt to taste

PREPARATION
Mix the soy sauce, sesame oil, honey, and vinegar in a bowl.
Stir the chopped beef cubes into the sauce and leave to marinate for 1 hour.

COOKING KOREAN STYLE BEEF SKEWERS IN AIR FRYER
Turn on the air fryer and set the temperature to 200°c. Skewer the pieces of beef on the skewers cut in half and place the skewers in the preheated fryer. Cook for about 10 minutes.

LAMB MEATBALLS

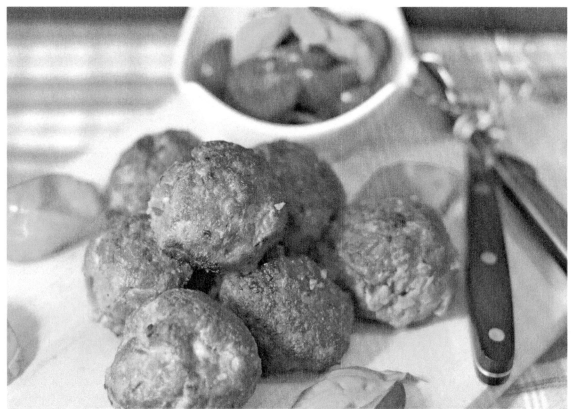

- **Preparation: 40 minutes**
- **Cooking time: 10 minutes**
- **Difficulty: Medium**
- **Servings: 3**

INGREDIENTS
- 450g Minced lamb
- Salt to taste
- 1g Black pepper
- 2g Freshly chopped mint
- 2g Ground cumin
- 3ml Hot sauce
- 1g Chilli powder
- 1 chopped Shallot
- 8g Chopped parsley
- 15ml Fresh lemon juice
- Lemon zest
- 10ml Olive oil

PREPARATION
Mix together the lamb, shallot, cumin, lemon juice, lemon zest, garlic, salt, pepper, hot sauce, chili powder and parsley. Shape the lamb mixture into 12 balls and chill in the refrigerator for 30 minutes.

COOKING LAMB MEATBALLS IN AIR FRYER
Turn on the air fryer and set to 180°c.
Coat the meatballs with olive oil and place them in the preheated fryer.
Set the time to 10 minutes and press start.

BACON IN AIR FRYER

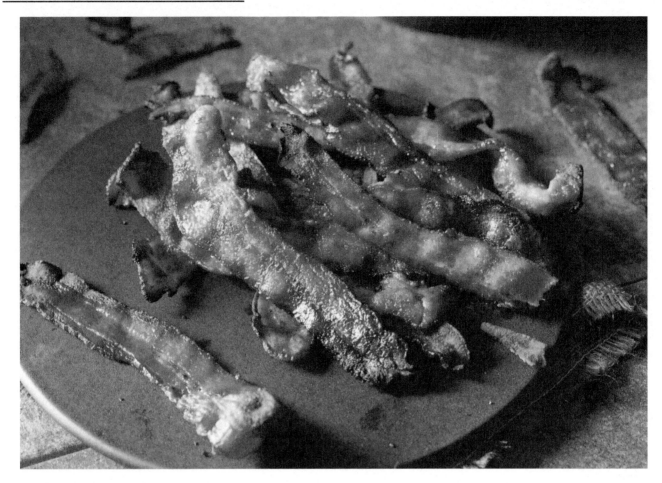

- **Preparation: 5 minutes**
- **Cooking time: 10 minutes**
- **Difficulty: Very easy**
- **Servings: 2**

INGREDIENTS
- 13g Cane sugar
- 5g Chilli powder
- 1g Ground cumin
- 1g Black pepper
- 4 slices of bacon

PREPARATION
Mix the toppings together until well combined.
Toss the bacon into the dressing until completely coated and set aside.

COOKING BACON IN AIR FRYER
Turn on the air fryer and adjust to 160°c. Place the bacon in the preheated fryer and cook for about 10 minutes.

PORK CHOPS

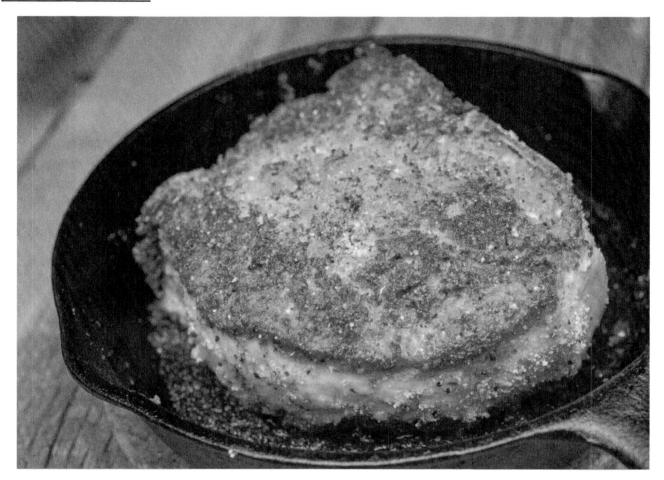

- **Preparation: 10 minutes**
- **Cooking time: 10 minutes**
- **Difficulty: Very easy**
- **Servings: 2**

INGREDIENTS
- 2 boneless Pork chops
- 15ml Vegetable oil
- 25g Dark cane sugar
- 6g Hungarian paprika
- 2g Ground mustard
- 2g Freshly ground black pepper
- 3g Onion powder
- 3g Garlic powder
- Salt and pepper to taste

PREPARATION
Cover the pork chops with oil.
Combine all the spices and season the pork chops, almost as if they were breaded.

COOKING PORK CHOPS IN AIR FRYER
Turn on the air fryer and set the temperature to 180°c. Place the pork chops in the preheated fryer and leave to cook for 10 minutes.

CAKE WITH HAM

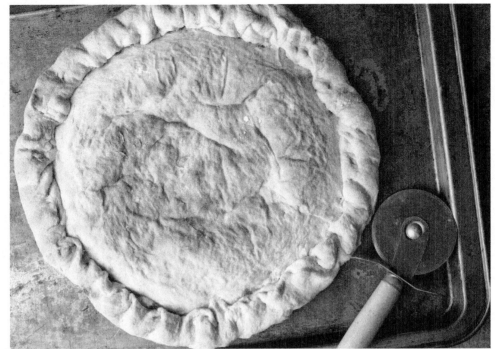

- **Preparation: 15 minutes**
- **Cooking time: 30 minutes**
- **Difficulty: Very easy**
- **Servings: 4**

INGREDIENTS
- 500g minced beef
- 1 Egg
- 100g Flour
- 3-4 Fresh basil leaves (finely chopped)
- 50g grated Parmesan cheese
- Salt and black pepper

For the stuffing
- 100g Cooked ham
- 3 slices Emmental cheese
- 4 tablespoons Tomato puree
- 150g provolone

PREPARATION
Add the egg, flour, chopped basil, parmesan, salt, and pepper to a bowl.
Knead with your hands in order to perfectly mix all the ingredients. If you prefer, you can use wet and squeezed stale breadcrumbs instead of flour.
Divide the dough into two equal parts. Line a 22cm mould with parchment paper and roll out the first half of the dough on the bottom. Stuff with sliced cooked ham, Emmental, and sliced provolone. Add basil leaves. Cover with the other half of the dough, adding a little at a time until it is completely closed. On the surface, add a few tablespoons of tomato sauce, basil, and cubes of provolone.

COOKING CAKE WITH HAM IN AIR FRYER
Use a mould that fits perfectly into the basket: place the mould in and cook at 180°c for about 20 minutes and a further 10 minutes at 200°c until completely browned.

PORK ROLLS WITH HAM

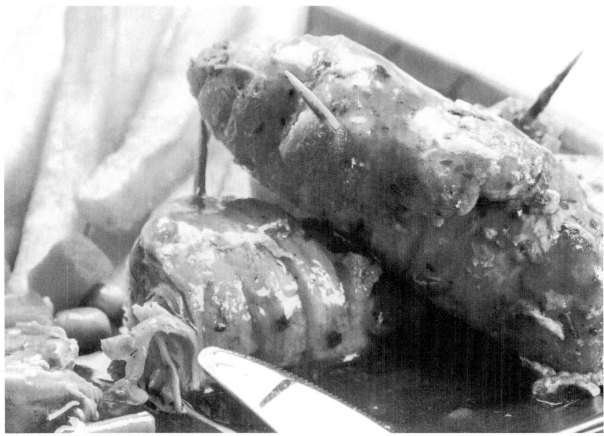

- **Preparation: 10 minutes**
- **Cooking time: 20 minutes**
- **Difficulty: Easy**
- **Servings: 4**

INGREDIENTS
- 6 pieces Sliced ham
- 1 Pork fillet (about 500g)
- 1g Black pepper
- 250g Spinach Leaves
- 4 slices Mozzarella
- 18g Dried cherry tomatoes
- 10ml EVO oil
- Salt to taste

PREPARATION
Season the inside of the pork rolls with salt and pepper. Arrange 3 pieces of ham on the parchment paper, slightly overlapping each other. Place 1 half of the pork on the ham and repeat with the other half. Place half the amount of spinach, cheese, and sliced sun-dried tomatoes on top of the pork, leaving a rim of about 15mm on all sides.
Roll tightly into the ham and tie it with kitchen twine to keep it closed.

COOKING PORK ROLLS WITH HAM IN A FRYER
Turn on the air fryer and set the temperature to 190°c.
Brush each wrapped pork with oil and put it in the preheated fryer, cooking for about 10 minutes. Leave the rolls to rest for another 10-12 minutes before serving.

FISH AND SEAFOOD RECIPES

FISH AND CHIPS

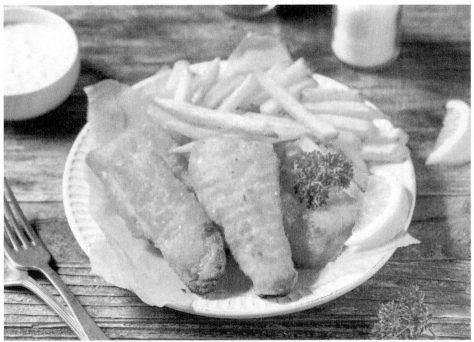

- **Preparation: 10 minutes**
- **Cooking time: 15 minutes**
- **Difficulty: Very easy**
- **Servings: 2**

INGREDIENTS
- 200g Cod fillet
- 1 Egg
- 300g Red potatoes
- 30g Breadcrumbs
- 1 tablespoon Vegetable oil
- Half a tablespoon Lemon juice
- Salt & Pepper if you prefer

PREPARATION
Cut the cod into equal parts and season it. For the dressing, you need to use lemon juice, salt, and pepper. Leave the seasoned fillet to rest for about five minutes.
Now, prepare the ingredients for the breading by beating the egg and placing the breadcrumbs on a serving dish. To bread the fillet, simply dip each piece of fish in the egg, covering the same piece with breadcrumbs after.
To prepare the potatoes, you need to peel the potatoes and cut them into sticks with a diameter of six or seven millimetres.

COOKING FISH AND CHIPS IN AIR FRYER
Preheat the fryer, setting the temperature to 180°c. Start cooking the fish fillet first and after 5 minutes, add the chips. The fish should be added to the basket of the oil-free fryer, along with the potatoes that is already frying, five minutes after the cooking starts.
Continue to fry the fish fillet and potatoes until they are golden in colour.

CROQUETTES OF COD

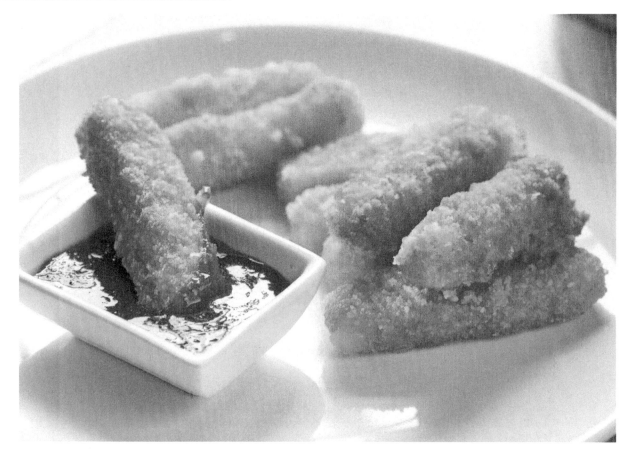

- **Preparation time: 10 minutes**
- **Cooking time: 8 minutes**
- **Difficulty: Very easy**
- **Servings: 4**

INGREDIENTS
- 450g Cod
- 30g All-purpose flour
- 7g Old Bay seasoning
- 2 Beaten eggs
- 180g Breadcrumbs

PREPARATION
Cut the fish into 40 x 15mm long strips. Mix together the Old Bay seasoning and the purpose flour in a plates. Cover each piece of fish with the seasoned flour, then dip into the eggs, and then the breadcrumbs.

COOKING COD CROQUETTES IN AIR FRYER
Turn on the air fryer and set the temperature to 180°c. Set the time to 8 minutes and press start. Shake the baskets halfway through cooking. Serve with tartar sauce.

SALMON WITH LEMON

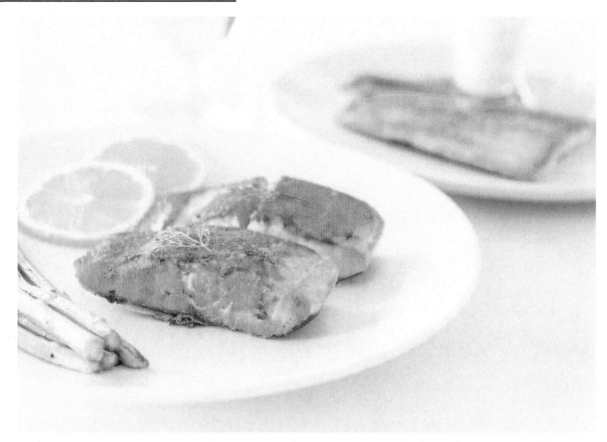

- **Preparation: 5 minutes**
- **Cooking time: 10 minutes**
- **Difficulty: Very easy**
- **Servings: 2**

INGREDIENTS
- 2 Salmon steaks
- Salt and pepper
- 30g Butter
- 30ml Fresh lemon juice
- 1 grated clove Garlic
- 5ml Worcestershire sauce
- Cooking spray

PREPARATION
Season the salmon to taste with salt and pepper.
Combine the lemon juice, garlic, and Worcestershire sauce and coat the salmon in the mixture. Divide the butter in two halves to place one half on each salmon steak.

COOKING SALMON WITH LEMON IN AIR FRYER
Turn on the air fryer and set the temperature to 180°c. Spray the preheated fryer baskets with cooking spray and put the fish inside.
Cook for about 10 minutes.

COUSCOUS SHRIMPS AND ZUCCHINI

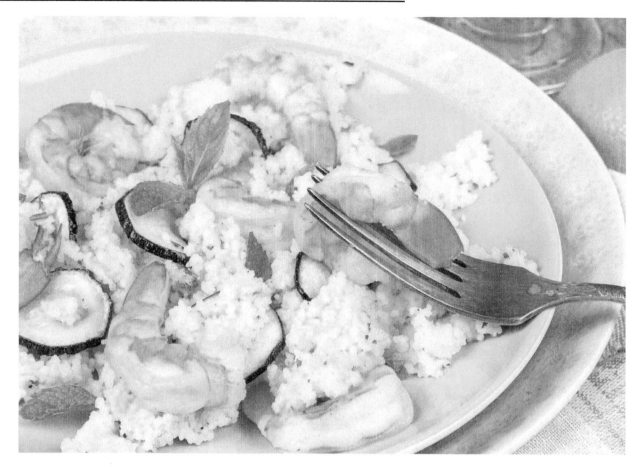

- **Preparation: 15 minutes**
- **Cooking time: 20 minutes**
- **Difficulty: Easy**
- **Servings: 2**

INGREDIENTS
- 180g Couscous
- 1 Courgette
- 150g Prawns
- 4 Mint leaves
- ½ Lemon
- 30ml Olive oil
- Salt to taste

PREPARATION
Cook the couscous following the instructions on the package.
Prepare the dressing by adding olive oil, lemon juice, and mint in a bowl. Save a small amount of the olive oil for later. Add salt to taste. Set it aside. Wash the courgettes and peel them, then slice them thinly with a knife. Clean the prawns and add them to the courgettes.

COOKING COUSCOUS SHRIMPS AND ZUCCHINI IN AIR FRYER
Place the shrimp and courgettes on the basket of the air fryer and season with a few drops of olive oil. Cook at 200°c for 8 minutes, turning them a couple of times. Season with salt, add to the couscous, and pour on your dressing, then toss and serve.

SLICED TUNA FISH

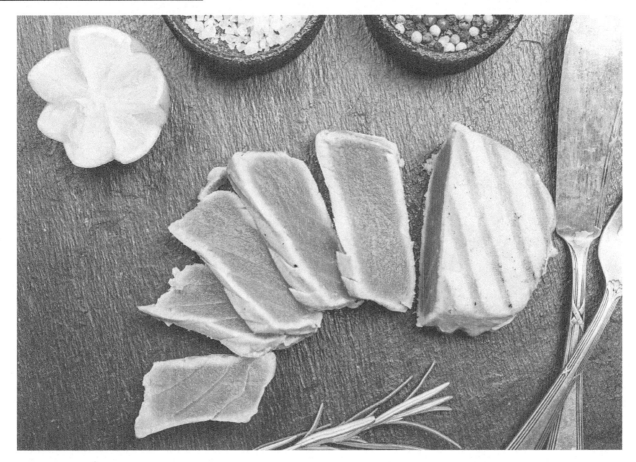

- **Preparation: 10 minutes**
- **Cooking time: 8 minutes**
- **Difficulty: Very easy**
- **Servings: 3**

INGREDIENTS
- 1 Tuna steak
- 25 ml Olive oil
- Salt to taste

PREPARATION
Place the tuna steak directly on the basket and brush on the olive oil on both sides.

COOKING SLICED TUNA IN AIR FRYER
Operate the air fryer at 180°c and cook the tuna for 4 minutes, then turn it gently, adding more olive oil. Then cook for another 4 minutes.
After cooking it, slice and serve.

SQUID RINGS

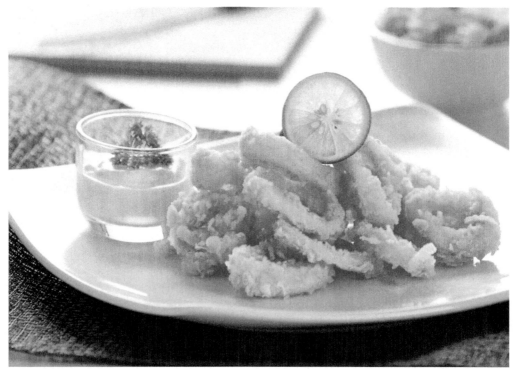

- **Preparation: 20 minutes**
- **Cooking time: 8 minutes**
- **Easy Difficulty**
- **Servings: 2**

INGREDIENTS
- 300g Fresh squid
- Seed oil (spray)
- 50g Semolina flour
- Salt to taste

PREPARATION
First of all, clean the squid.
Rinse them under running water. Detach the head by eliminating the whole central body, keep it aside. Clean internally, removing the entrails and rinsing well. Then cut them into rings and set aside to dry. Put the flour in a plastic bag and toss the squid rings in it.

COOKING SQUID RINGS IN AIR FRYER
Put a little oil in the basket and place the squid in it, not overlapping them: rather, cook them in portions if you have to.
Spray the squid with a few puffs of oil using an oil spray. Cook at 200°c for 7-8 minutes, depending on the size and thickness of the squid.

SALMON GRATIN

- **Preparation: 10 minutes**
- **Cooking time: 8 minutes**
- **Difficulty: Very easy**
- **Servings: 2**

INGREDIENTS

- 2 Salmon steaks
- 100g Wholemeal breadcrumbs
- ½ Lemon (juice and zest)
- 5g Aromatic herbs of your choice
- Salt to taste
- Oil

PREPARATION

Place the breadcrumbs in a bowl. Flavour with chopped aromatic herbs and lemon zest. Squeeze lemon juice over salmon, coating it. Then, dip the salmon steak in the breadcrumbs and coat it evenly.

COOKING IN AIR FRYER

Place the salmon directly on the basket of the air fryer at 180°c. Cook for about 8 minutes, turning it halfway through cooking.

BACON SHRIMPS

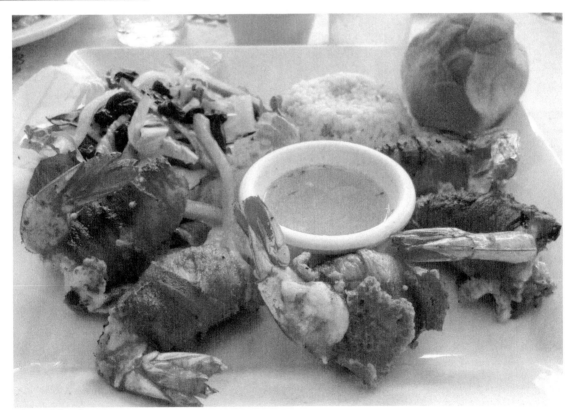

- **Preparation: 10 minutes**
- **Cooking time: 18 minutes**
- **Difficulty: Easy**
- **Servings: 4**

INGREDIENTS

- 16 Peeled giant prawns
- 3g Garlic powder
- 2g Paprika
- 2g Onion powder
- 1g Ground black pepper
- 8 strips Bacon

PREPARATION

Cut each of your bacon strips into two. Season the jumbo prawns with all the spices, wrap each one of them with bacon and hold them with a toothpick.

BACON SHRIMPS COOKING IN AIR FRYER

Turn on the air fryer and set the temperature to 160°c.
Press start and allow to cook for 18 minutes. At the end of cooking, set aside.

FISH BURGER

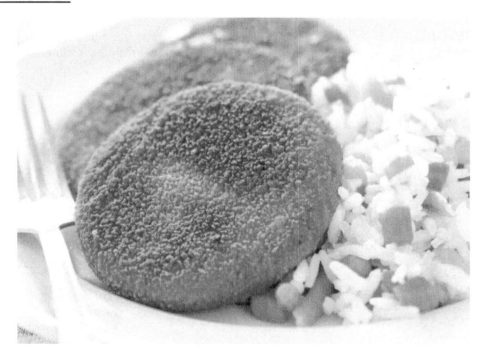

- **Cooking: 15 minutes**
- **Preparation: 5 minutes**
- **Difficulty: Easy**
- **Serves: 4 people**

INGREDIENTS
- 100g Stale bread
- 400g Swordfish cut into pieces
- 200g Salmon
- 20g Apple cider vinegar
- 20g Lemon juice
- Salt and pepper
- Parsley

PREPARATION

Crumb the stale bread with a food processor. Add the lemon, vinegar, swordfish, and mix for a few more seconds, until you get a thick and creamy consistency. Divide the mixture into 4-5 parts. Shape into meatballs and then press until you get the classic hamburger shape.

COOKING FISH BURGER IN THE AIR FRYER

Cook in an air fryer at 180°c for 15 minutes.

SWORDFISH GRATIN

• **Preparation: 10 minutes**
• **Cooking time: 10 minutes**
• **Difficulty: Medium**
• **Servings: 2**

INGREDIENTS
• 4 slices Swordfish
• 1 glass White wine
• 1 sprig Rosemary
• 2 cloves Garlic
• 4 slices Stale bread
• Salt and pepper
• 10g Chives
• 1 pinch f Paprika
• 25ml Olive oil
• 6 tablespoons Almonds

PREPARATION
Remove the swordfish from the marinating liquid and transfer it to a plate. If you are using non-marinated frozen swordfish, it will only need to be gratinated once thawed.
Pour the bread into a food processor, add the almonds, salt, pepper, garlic powder (or a clove of fresh garlic), three tablespoons of olive oil, and a pinch of paprika, and chop everything. Salt the slices of swordfish and then distribute the sauce on each slice.

COOKING SWORDFISH GRATIN IN AIR FRYER
Arrange the slices of swordfish au gratin on the grill of the air fryer.
Cook the swordfish at a temperature of 160°c for about 10 minutes.

FRIED MUSSELS

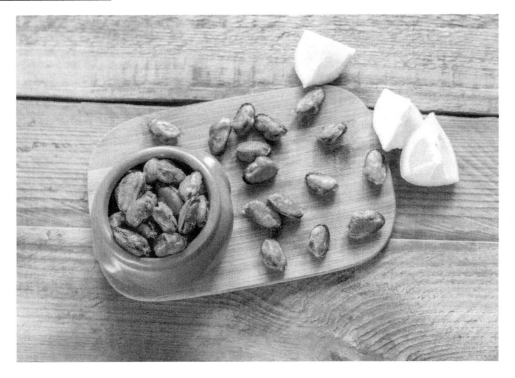

- **Cooking: 10 minutes**
- **Preparation: 10 minutes**
- **Difficulty: Easy**
- **Servings: 4 people**

INGREDIENTS
- 1kg Mussels
- 1 Egg
- 2 tablespoons Flour
- 2 tablespoons Parsley
- 2 tablespoons Mineral water
- 1 clove Garlic
- Seed oil
- Salt and pepper

PREPARATION
Wash the mussels by putting them in water and eliminating those already open. Clean the mussels thoroughly, put them in a pan, cover and cook until they open, stirring occasionally. Prepare the batter, mixing the flour with the egg, the chopped parsley, garlic, salt, and pepper, and finally, the cold mineral water. Remove the mussels from their shells and dip them in the batter.

COOKING IN AIR FRYER
Cook in the preheated air fryer at 180°c for 7-10 minutes. Turn during cooking.

CATFISH

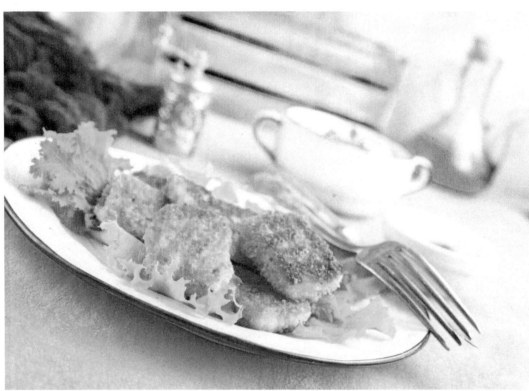

- **Preparation: 15 minutes**
- **Cooking: 20 minutes**
- **Difficulty: Easy**
- **Servings: 4**

INGREDIENTS
- 600g Catfish fillet
- 100g Flour
- 3g Cayenne pepper
- 4g Onion powder
- 4g Garlic powder
- 3g Sweet paprika
- 20ml Extra virgin olive oil and salt

PREPARATION
Rinse the fillets under running water and dry them. Cut them into 3-4 cm pieces. In a plastic bag, pour the flour with the spices and shake to mix. Add the freshly cut morsels and shake the bag again, making them cover evenly.

COOKING IN FRYER
Grease the fryer basket and arrange the catfish. Cook them at 210°c for 20 minutes, checking the cooking often and shaking the basket.

GRILLED FISH TACOS

- **Preparation: 10 minutes**
- **Cooking time: 8 minutes**
- **Difficulty: Easy**
- **Servings: 4**

INGREDIENTS
- 450g sliced Tilapia
- 100g Flour
- 1g Ground cumin
- 1g Chilli powder
- 2g Garlic powder
- 1 Onion powder
- 3g Salt
- 1g Black pepper
- Lime wedges and taco shells for serving

PREPARATION
Cut the tilapia into strips.
Mix together the flour and seasonings in a deep plate.
Coat the fish strips with the mixture and set aside in the fridge.

COOKING GRILLED FISH TACOS IN AIR FRYER
Turn on the air fryer and set the temperature to 180°c.
Generously spray the coated fish with cooking spray and place it in the preheated fryer.
Adjust the time to 10 minutes and press start.
Flip the fish halfway through cooking.
Serve the fish with lime wedges.

SIDES RECIPES

BACON, EGG, AND SPINACH TARTLETS

- **Preparation: 5 minutes**
- **Cooking time: 15 minutes**
- **Difficulty Very easy**
- **Servings: 3**

INGREDIENTS
- 3 Eggs
- 6 slices Bacon
- 60g Spinach washed
- 100ml Cream
- 20g Grated parmesan cheese
- Salt and pepper to taste

PREPARATION
Prepare the moulds of about 10 cm in diameter and add an egg in each of them. Cook the bacon in a skillet until crisp, about 5 minutes. Add the spinach and cook for another 2 minutes.
Mix the cream and the grated parmesan. Cook for 2 to 3 minutes.
Pour the cream mixture over the eggs.

COOKING IN AIR FRYER
Turn on the air fryer and set the temperature to 180°c.
Place the moulds in the preheated air fryer and cook for 15 minutes at 170°c. Season with pepper and salt.

GRATIN BROCCOLI

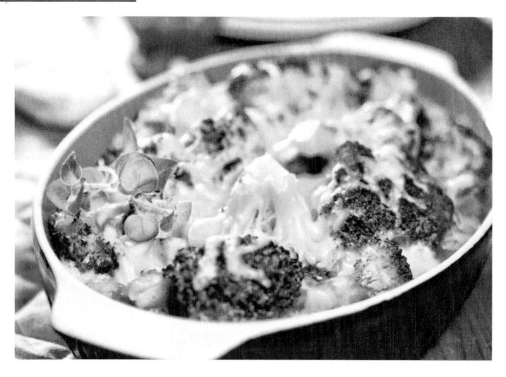

- **Preparation: 15 minutes**
- **Cooking time: 30 minutes**
- **Difficulty Very easy**
- **Servings: 4**

INGREDIENTS
- Broccoli (about 400g)
- 1 clove Garlic
- 2 slices of Bread
- Olive oil
- Chilli pepper
- Fine salt

PREPARATION
Clean the broccoli by removing the stem, i.e., keeping the florets. Steam the broccoli in salted water, according to the traditional method.
When it is cooked, drain it, and remove the excess water. Cut the bread into tiny cubes or crumble it in a processor. Season it with herbs. In a pan, fry the garlic with the chilli and olive oil. Add the broccoli and bread and sauté for a few minutes to flavour.

COOKING BROCCOLI GRATIN IN AIR FRYER
After a few minutes, put everything in a baking dish and brown in an air fryer at 200°c for 5 minutes.

POTATOES WITH SPECK, WALNUTS, AND GORGONZOLA

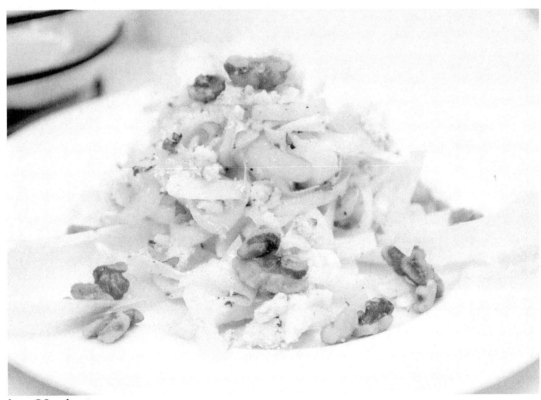

- **Preparation: 30 minutes**
- **Cooking time: 40 minutes**
- **Difficulty: Very easy**
- **Servings: 2**

INGREDIENTS
- 3-4 Potatoes
- 100g Speck
- 80g Gorgonzola
- 10 Walnuts
- Salt and pepper

PREPARATION
Boil the potatoes in salted water. When they are soft inside, drain and let them cool.

Put the potatoes in a bowl, mash them with a fork to purée them. Add the salt and pepper, the sliced speck, and the gorgonzola.

Add the crumbled walnuts and mix to mix all the ingredients well. You can add aromatic herbs or a little olive oil.

COOKING IN THE AIR FRYER
In an air fryer, place a pan with the potatoes directly on the basket of the air fryer and cook them at 200°c for about 8-10 minutes.

VEGAN BURGER WITH POTATOES AND COURGETTES

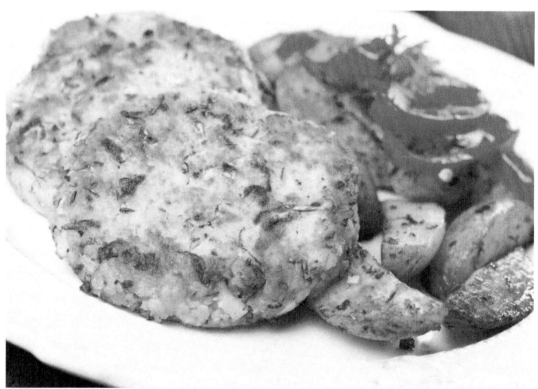

- **Preparation: 20 minutes**
- **Cooking time: 15 minutes**
- **Difficulty: Very easy**
- **Servings: 4**

INGREDIENTS
- 2 Courgettes
- 3 Potatoes
- 1 Egg
- 100g Mozzarella
- 50gf Flour

- 30g Breadcrumbs
- 2 tablespoons Parmesan cheese
- 1 Egg for breading
- Salt, pepper, and oil

PREPARATION

Prepare the potatoes, wash them, and grate them by hand. Also grate the courgettes in the same way as the potatoes. Combine the courgettes and potatoes in a bowl, add the whole egg, parmesan, salt, and pepper, and flour and breadcrumbs little by little, until the mixture is soft and workable, to be able to mould your hamburgers.

Using a pastry cutter placed on baking paper, fill the bottom then stuff with mozzarella. Seal with more of the mixture.

COOKING VEGAN BURGER WITH POTATOES AND COURGETTES IN AIR FRYER

Arrange the burgers on pieces of parchment paper and sprinkle them with olive oil. Cook them at 200°c for the first 5 minutes, then you can remove the parchment paper, turn them, and proceed with cooking for another 5 minutes.

<u>CUTLET OF AUBERGINES</u>

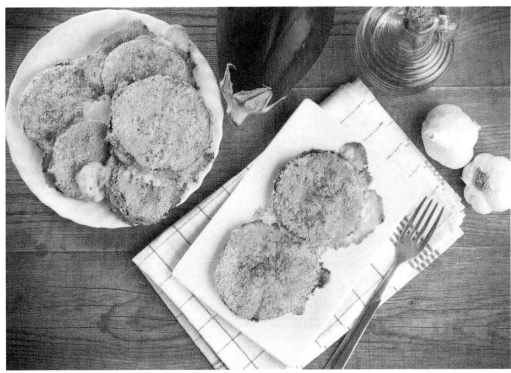

- **Preparation: 10 minutes**
- **Cooking time: 10 minutes**
- **Difficulty: Very easy**
- **Servings: 2**

INGREDIENTS

- 1 Beaten egg
- 15ml Milk
- 100g Breadcrumbs
- 1g Black pepper
- 1 Eggplant cut into slices
- 60g Flour

- Olive oil (spray)
- Salt and pepper

PREPARATION

Whisk together the egg and milk. Combine the breadcrumbs, salt, and pepper in a separate dish. Cut the aubergines into slices. Cover the eggplant slices with flour, then dip them in the egg and then in the breadcrumbs.

COOKING IN AIR FRYER

Turn on the air fryer and set the temperature to 200°c.
Spritz each side of the eggplant slices with the olive oil spray.
Preheat the air fryer at 200°c and cook the aubergine for 10 minutes, flipping them halfway through the cooking.

CROQUETTES OF MOZZARELLA

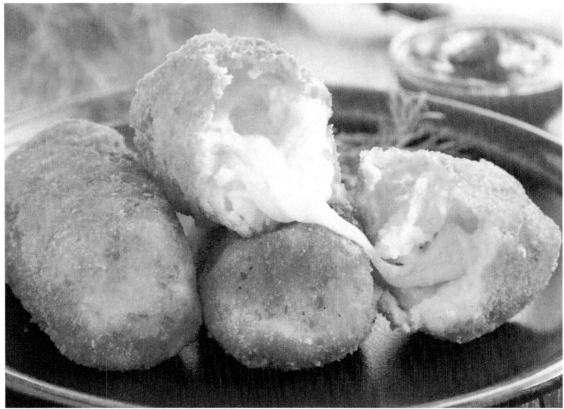

- **Preparation: 10 minutes**
- **Cooking time: 10 minutes**
- **Difficulty: Very easy**
- **Servings: 3**

INGREDIENTS
- 6 Mozzarellas
- 20g Flour
- 3g Corn starch
- 3g Salt
- 1g Black pepper
- 2 eggs (beaten)
- 15ml Milk
- 50g Breadcrumbs
- 1 pinch Dried parsley

44

PREPARATION

Mix together the flour, corn starch, salt, and pepper in a bowl. Whisk the eggs and milk together in a separate bowl. Combine the breadcrumbs and parsley flakes in an additional bowl.
Cover each mozzarella with flour, then dip it in the egg and roll it in breadcrumbs.

COOKING MOZZARELLA CROQUETTES IN AIR FRYER

Turn on the air fryer and set the temperature to 170°c.
Place the mozzarella croquettes in the preheated fryer. Set the time to 8 minutes.
Shake the baskets halfway through cooking. Serve with your favourite sauce.

STUFFED CHAMPIGNON

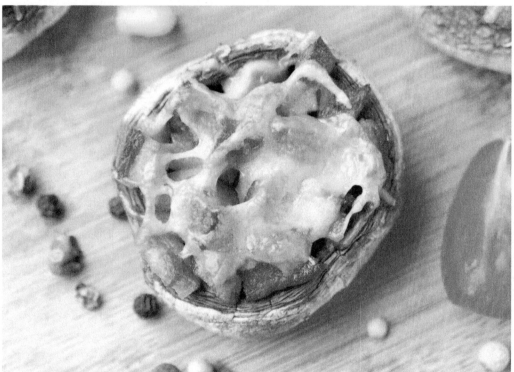

- **Preparation: 20 minutes**
- **Cooking time: 15 minutes**
- **Difficulty: Very easy**
- **Servings: 2**

INGREDIENTS

- 6 Champignon mushrooms
- 20ml Olive oil
- 1 minced Clove of garlic
- 100g Sausage
- 15g Breadcrumbs
- 50g Grated mozzarella
- 20g Grated parmesan cheese
- 4g Chopped parsley
- Salt and pepper to taste

PREPARATION

Remove the mushroom stems from the caps. Chop the stems and set them aside. Scoop out the inside of the mushrooms to make more room for the filling. Heat a pan with garlic and oil over medium heat.

Add 15ml of olive oil and chopped mushroom stems, then cook for 5 minutes.

Add the sausage and cook until browned, about 5 minutes, and then set aside. Allow it to rest for about three minutes, then into pieces.

Mix the sausage with the breadcrumbs, mozzarella (half), parmesan, and parsley.

Season to taste with pepper and salt.

Fill the mushrooms and dress them with more mozzarella.

COOKING STUFFED CHAMPIGNON IN AIR FRYER

Turn on the air fryer and set the temperature to 180°c.

Place the stuffed mushrooms in the preheated air fryer.

Cook the mushrooms at 180°c for 15 minutes.

AUBERGINES WITH PARMIGIANO

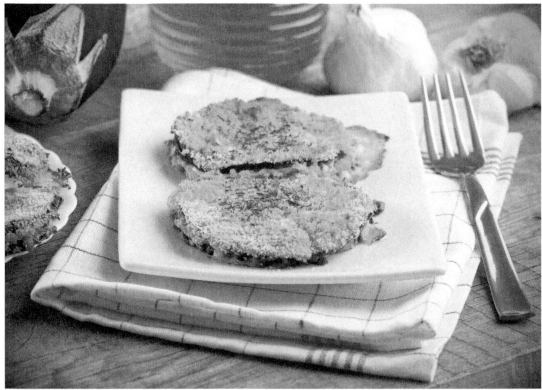

- **Preparation: 20 minutes**
- **Cooking time: 15 minutes**
- **Difficulty: Very easy**
- **Servings: 2**

INGREDIENTS
- 1 Eggplant (about 500g)
- 50g Parmesan breading
- 20ml Olive oil
- 2g Fine salt

PREPARATION

Wash the eggplant and dry it with a clean cloth or kitchen roll. Cut it in half lengthwise without removing the middle. With a knife, cut it into slices delicately lengthwise. Spray the surface with a little oil. Prepare the parmesan breading for the gratin and sprinkle it all over the surface of each slice.

COOKING AUBERGINES WITH PARMIGIANO IN AIR FRYER
Place the aubergines on the basket. Spray the surface with olive oil using an oil spray bottle. Cook them at 150°c for about 12 minutes. Then, for the last minutes 3 minutes, when cooked, increase to 200° to finish the gratin.

ROAST PUMPKIN

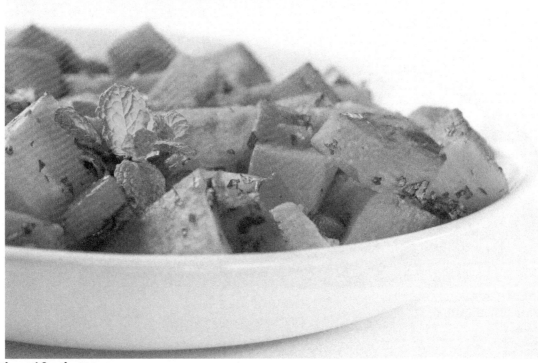

- **Preparation: 10 minutes**
- **Cooking time: 12 minutes**
- **Difficulty Very easy**
- **Servings: 3**

INGREDIENTS
- 1 Orange pumpkin
- 15ml Olive oil
- 1g Thyme leaves
- Salt
- Black pepper

PREPARATION
Cut the pumpkin into cubes of about 4cm.
Cover the pumpkin cubes with olive oil and season with pepper, thyme, and salt. Add the seasoned pumpkin to the preheated fryer.

COOKING ROAST PUMPKIN IN AIR FRYER
Turn on the air fryer and set the temperature to 170°c.
Be sure to shake the basket halfway through cooking. Drizzle with olive oil when cooked and serve.

ONION RINGS

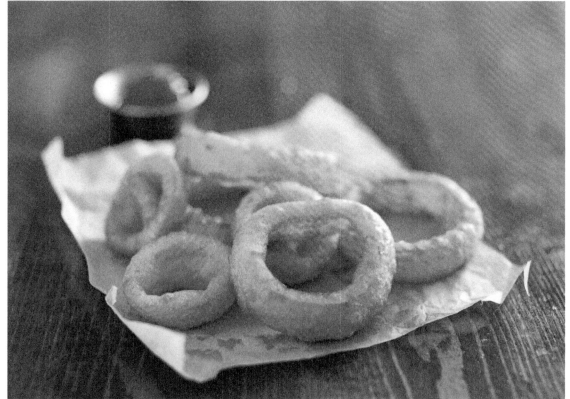

- **Preparation: 10 minutes**
- **Cooking time: 20 minutes**
- **Difficulty: Very easy**
- **Servings 2**

INGREDIENTS
- 1 Onion
- 80g Breadcrumbs
- 2g Smoked paprika
- Salt
- 2 Eggs
- 100ml Buttermilk
- 60g Flour
- Cooking spray

PREPARATION
Cut the onion into 12mm thick slices and separate the layers into rings. In a bowl, combine paprika, salt and breadcrumbs, then set aside. Beat the eggs and the buttermilk together until completely blended. Dip each onion ring in the flour, eggs mixture, and then the breadcrumb mixture.

COOKING ONION RINGS IN AIR FRYER
Turn on the air fryer and set the temperature to 190°c. Generously spray the onion rings with cooking spray. Place the onion rings in a single layer in the baskets of the preheated fryer and batch cook at 190°c for 10 minutes until golden brown. Serve with sauce.

POTATO WEDGES

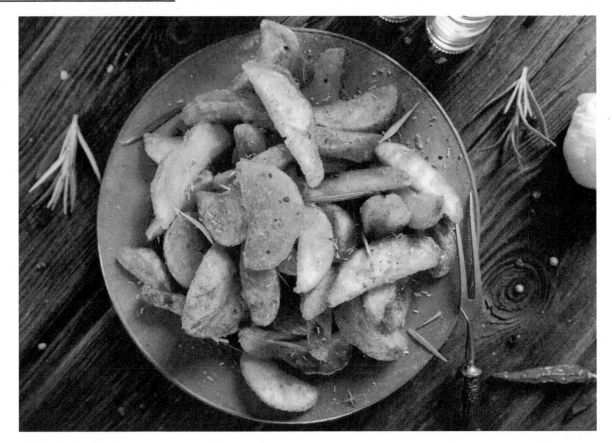

- **Preparation: 5 minutes**
- **Cooking time: 20 minutes**
- **Difficulty: Very easy**
- **Servings: 4**

INGREDIENTS
- 2 large Potatoes
- 20ml Olive oil
- 3g Garlic powder
- 1 teaspoon Onion powder
- 3g Salt
- 1g Black pepper
- 5g grated Parmesan cheese
- Ketchup or mayonnaise for serving

PREPARATION
Cut the potatoes into wedges.
Toss the potatoes in a bowl with the olive oil and all the seasoning including the parmesan.

COOKING POTATO WEDGES IN AIR FRYER
Turn on the air fryer and set the temperature to 200°c.
Select French Fries on the air fryer, set the timer to 20 minutes and press start.
Shake the baskets halfway through cooking. Serve with ketchup or mayonnaise.

FRIED AVOCADO

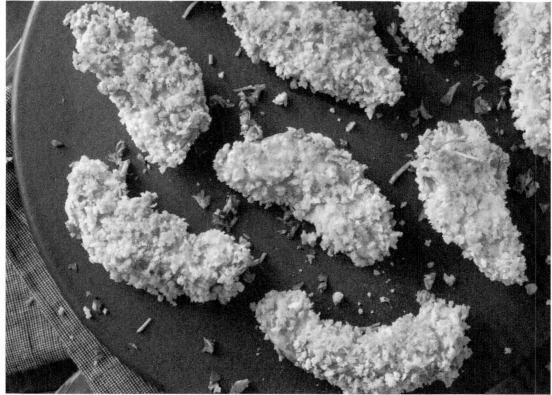

- **Preparation: 20 minutes**
- **Cooking time: 10 minutes**
- **Difficulty: Very easy**
- **Servings: 2**

INGREDIENTS
- 2 Avocados cut into wedges
- 50g Breadcrumbs
- 2g Garlic powder
- 2g Onion powder
- 1g Smoked paprika
- 1g Cayenne pepper
- Salt and pepper to taste
- 60g Flour
- 2 Beaten Eggs
- Cooking spray
- Ketchup or mayonnaise for serving

PREPARATION
Cut the avocados into 25 mm thick wedges. Combine the onion powder with breadcrumbs, garlic powder, paprika, pepper and salt in a bowl.
Dip the avocado wedges into the flour then the beaten eggs and roll it in the breadcrumb mixture.

COOKING FRIED AVOCADO IN AIR FRYER
Turn on the air fryer and set the temperature to 200°c.
Place the fried avocados in the baskets of the preheated fryer, spray with cooking spray and cook at 200°c for 10 minutes. Flip the avocados halfway through cooking. Serve with ketchup or mayonnaise for dipping.

FRIED COURGETTE

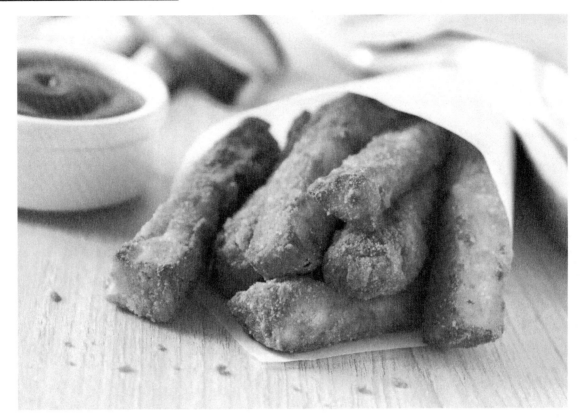

- **Preparation: 10 minutes**
- **Cooking time: 10 minutes**
- **Difficulty: Very easy**
- **Servings 4**

INGREDIENTS
- 1 Medium courgette
- 60g Flour
- 12g Salt
- 2g Black pepper
- 2 Eggs, beaten
- 15ml Milk
- 85g seasoned Breadcrumbs
- 25g of grated Parmesan cheese
- Non-stick cooking spray

PREPARATION
Cut the courgettes into 20mm thick strips. Mix the flours, pepper and salt in a dish. Whisk the milk and the eggs together in a separate dish. Combine the breadcrumbs and parmesan in another dish.
Cover each piece of courgette with flour, then dip them in the egg, roll in the breadcrumbs and set aside.

COOKING FRIED ZUCCHINI IN AIR FRYER
Turn on the air fryer and set the temperature to 175°c.
Place the courgettes in the preheated fryer and spray with non-stick cooking spray, set the time to 10 minutes and press start. Shake the baskets halfway through cooking.

ROASTED PEPPERS

- Preparation: 5 minutes
- Cooking time: 20 minutes
- Difficulty: Very easy
- Servings: 3

INGREDIENTS
- 3 Peppers
- Salt and pepper

PREPARATION
Wash the peppers well, choosing the perfect ones without bruises.
Dry them carefully by dabbing the surface. There is no need to cut them or remove the stalk and seeds.

COOKING ROASTED PEPPERS IN AIR FRYER
Place the peppers directly on the basket of the air fryer. Operate and cook at 200°c for 20 minutes, turning them a couple of times in order to change sides. Season with salt and pepper and serve.

POTATO ROLLS

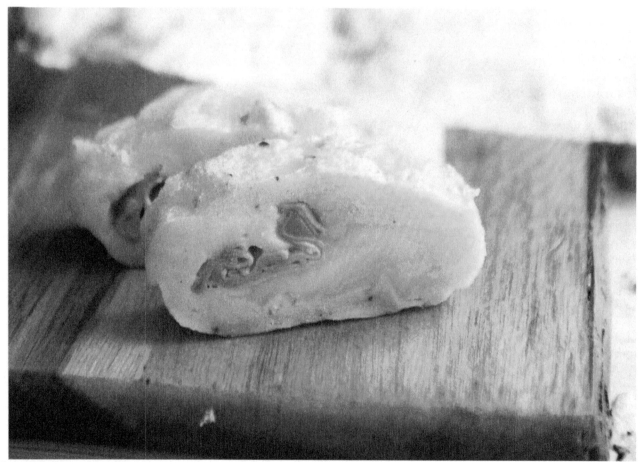

- **Preparation: 40 minutes**
- **Cooking time: 15 minutes**
- **Difficulty Very easy**
- **Servings: 4**

INGREDIENTS
- 250g boiled Potatoes
- 110g Flour
- 30g grated Parmesan
- 1 Egg
- 1 pinch Fine Salt
- 30g Flour

For the stuffing
- 150g cooked Ham
- 150g Cheese (sliced)

PREPARATION
Boil the potatoes in salted water. Drain them when they are cooked. With a potato masher, mash then until they are soft. Put the mashed potatoes in a bowl, add the egg, a pinch of salt, and ¾ of the flour. Knead until the mixture is well combined.

Form a loaf and roll it out with a rolling pin, sprinkling it little by little with flour, on the surface also. Form a rectangle and stuff it with sliced ham and cheese.

Roll and seal the edges well so that the filling does not come out during cooking.

COOKING IN AIR FRYER
Place the potato roll on the basket with parchment paper and sprinkle it with a drizzle of oil. Cook it at 180°c for about 15 minutes, turning it halfway through cooking.

ROASTED AUBERGINES

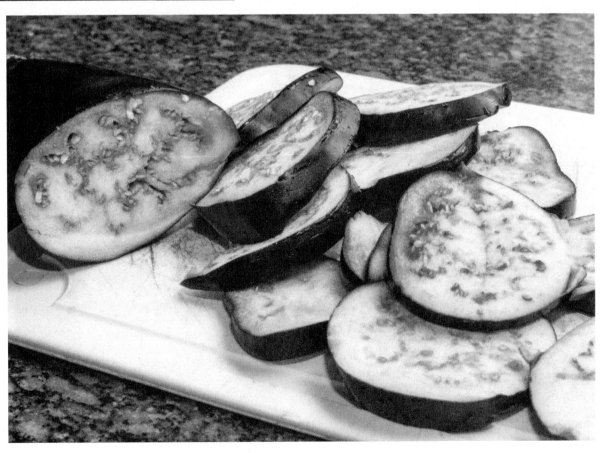

- **Preparation: 10 minutes**
- **Cooking time: 10 minutes**
- **Difficulty: Very easy**
- **Servings: 2**

INGREDIENTS
- 1 Eggplant
- 30ml Olive oil
- Salt
- 2g Garlic powder
- 1g Black pepper
- 1 Onion powder
- 1g Ground cumin

PREPARATION
Cut the aubergines into slices of about 1 cm thick. Wisk the seasoning with the olive oil in a large bowl and spread the mixture on top of the eggplant.

COOKING IN A FRYER
Turn on the air fryer and set the temperature to 200°c.
Place the aubergines in the air fryer and cook for 10 minutes.

ROASTED CAULIFLOWERS

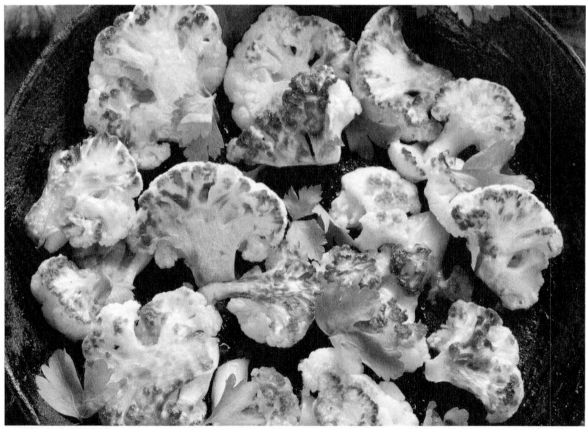

- **Preparation: 5 minutes**
- **Cooking time: 10 minutes**
- **Difficulty: Very easy**
- **Servings: 3**

INGREDIENTS
- 300g Cauliflower florets
- 10ml Olive oil
- 3g Salt
- 1g Black pepper

PREPARATION
Put the cauliflower florets in a bowl, add a drizzle of olive oil and season with salt and pepper evenly.

COOKING IN A FRYER
Turn on the air fryer and set the temperature to 150°c.
Add the cauliflower to the preheated air fryer and cook for about 10 minutes.

SNACKS AND APPETIZERS

AUBERGINE FAGOTTINI ALLA PIZZAIOLA

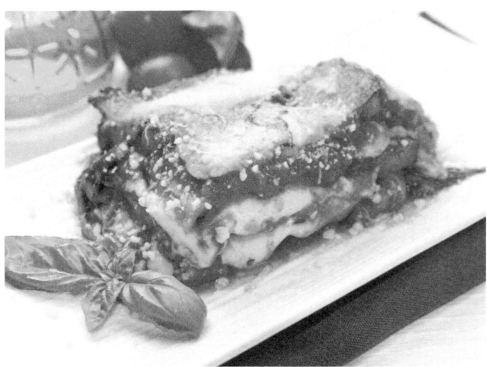

- **Preparation: 20 minutes**
- **Cooking time: 15 minutes**
- **Difficulty: Easy**
- **Servings: 4**

INGREDIENTS
- 4 Aubergines
- 300ml Tomato puree
- 500g Milk ricotta
- 40g grated Parmesan cheese
- 4-5 fresh Basil leaves
- 150g Smoked cheese
- Salt
- 30ml Olive oil

PREPARATION
Wash the aubergines, peel them, and cut them into thin slices.
Grill them on a hot plate and bake at 200°c for 15 minutes. Prepare the filling: put the drained ricotta in a bowl, add the parmesan, half the diced smoked, fine salt, and chopped basil.
Mix well to combine all the ingredients and make the ricotta creamy.
Prepare the bundles: lay 4 slices of aubergine crossing them two by two. Add the filling with a spoon and close the bundle.
Prepare the tomato: add the puree in a bowl, season with a little oil, salt, and fresh basil.
Put a few tablespoons of tomato puree on the bottom of a baking dish, place the bundles and cover them with sauce, diced smoked cheese, and grated parmesan.

COOKING IN AIR FRYER
Cook the bundles at 200°c for 10 minutes, check that they are cooked through; otherwise, continue for another 5-10 minutes.

CHEESE MUFFIN

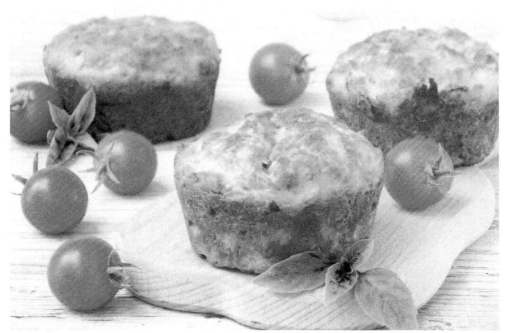

- **Preparation: 10 minutes**
- **Cooking time: 15 minutes**
- **Difficulty Very easy**
- **Servings: 6**

INGREDIENTS
- 60g Flour
- 80g Corn flour
- 40g White sugar
- 6g Salt
- 7g Baking powder
- 120ml Milk
- 45g melted Butter
- 1 Egg
- 150g Corn
- 3 chopped Shallots
- 120g grated Cheddar cheese
- Non-stick cooking spray

PREPARATION
Combine flour, corn flour, sugar, salt, and yeast in a bowl and mix.
Whisk together milk, butter, and eggs until well combined.
Combine both wet and dry mixture together, add the corn along with shallots and the cheddar.

COOKING CHEESE MUFFIN IN AIR FRYER
Turn on the air fryer and set the temperature to 160°c with the bread settings.
Add the muffins to the preheated fryer and cook for 15 minutes.
Serve the muffins with butter or as they are.

ROASTED CORN

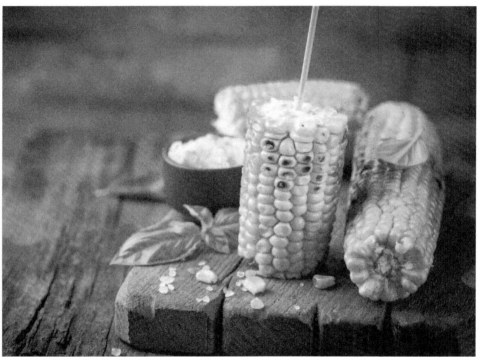

• **Preparation: 5 minutes**
• **Cooking time: 10 minutes**
• **Difficulty: Very easy**
• **Servings: 1**

INGREDIENTS
• 1 Corn cob
• 15g melted Butter
• Salt to taste

PREPARATION
Brush the melted butter all over the corn and season with salt.

COOKING ROASTED CORN IN AIR FRYER
Turn on the air fryer and set the temperature to 170°c.
Select the Root Vegetables setting, set the timer to 10 minutes and press start.
Flip the plus halfway through cooking.

CORDON BLEU

• **Preparation: 15 minutes**
• **Cooking time: 12 minutes**
• **Difficulty: Very easy**
• **Servings: 2**

INGREDIENTS

- 4 slices Veal
- 2 slices smoked Cheese
- 2 slices cooked Ham
- 3 medium Tarallo
- 1 Egg
- 1 teaspoon Olive oil
- Fine salt

PREPARATION

Chop the Tarallo with a mixer in a coarse way: you do not want it to be too fine, but more of a delicious grain.
Stuff half of the veal slices with cooked ham, smoked cheese, then more cooked ham. Cover with another slice of meat, taking care to seal the edges well. Beat the egg with a pinch of salt. Dip the cordon bleu and gently make sure that it is completely covered by the egg. Dip it in the Tarallo breading and press it so that it adheres perfectly.

COOKING CORDON BLEU IN AIR FRYER

Place the cordon bleu on parchment paper, then and directly on the fryer basket. Bake at 200°c for 10-12 minutes until golden brown. You can remove the parchment paper after 2-3 minutes.

BREAD CROUTONS

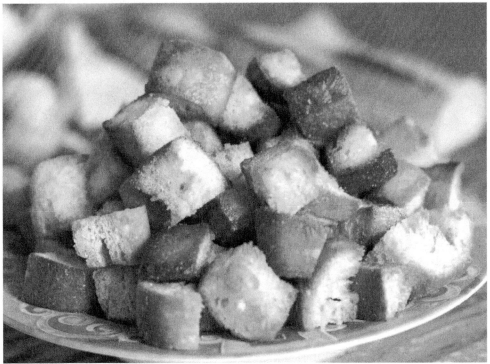

- **Preparation: 10 minutes**
- **Cooking time: 5 minutes**
- **Difficulty: Very easy**
- **Servings: 3**

INGREDIENTS

- 200g Bread
- Aromatic herbs (thyme, rosemary, sage, oregano)
- Salt to taste
- 50ml Olive oil

PREPARATION

Cut the bread into cubes, making sure they are roughly the same size. You can use both the crumb and the outer crust to make croutons, depending on your preferences.

Place the pieces of bread in a bowl and season them with the salt and chopped aromatic herbs (thyme, rosemary, sage, and oregano).

Mix so that they are perfectly flavoured and place them on the air fryer's basket.

COOKING BREAD CROUTONS IN AIR FRYER

Operate the air fryer at 200°c and cook for 5-6 minutes, until they are golden and crispy as desired.

CHESTNUTS

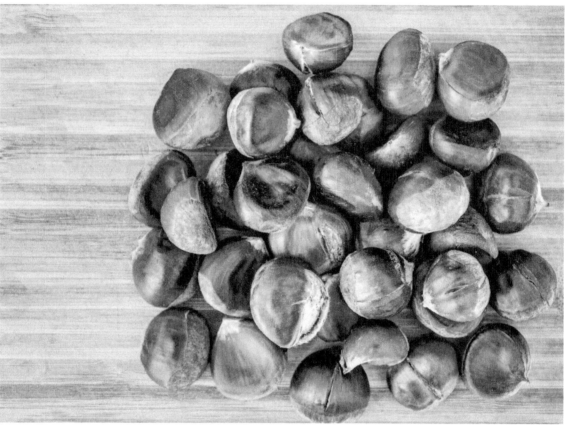

- **Preparation: 10 minutes**
- **Cooking time: 20 minutes**
- **Difficulty: Very easy**
- **Servings: 3**

INGREDIENTS
- 30 Chestnuts

PREPARATION

Carve the chestnuts on the surface from the rounded part: you can decide to make a single cut or a crosscut, which is more attractive because it opens wider during cooking.

COOKING CHESTNUTS IN AIR FRYER

Arrange the chestnuts directly on the basket, with the incised and rounded part upwards. Operate the fryer at 180°c and cook for 15-20 minutes.

PUMPKIN AND SAUSAGE

- **Preparation: 10 minutes**
- **Cooking time: 8 minutes**
- **Difficulty: Very easy**
- **Servings: 2**

INGREDIENTS
- 200g Sausage
- 300g Pumpkin
- 2 teaspoons Olive oil
- Fine salt
- Oregano
- Herbs

PREPARATION
Peel the pumpkin, getting rid of the pulp, then cut it into cubes of about 1-2 cm. Cut the sausage into rather small pieces and place them together with the pumpkin in a bowl. Season with a teaspoon of oil, salt, and oregano or your favourite aromatic herbs. Mix well to blend the flavours and distribute the herbs evenly.

COOKING PUMPKIN AND SAUSAGE IN AIR FRYER
Place the pumpkin and sausage directly on the air fryer basket without moulds or parchment paper.
Operate the air fryer at 180°c and cook for 8 minutes or the time necessary to make it cook through.

DONUTS WITH SUGAR

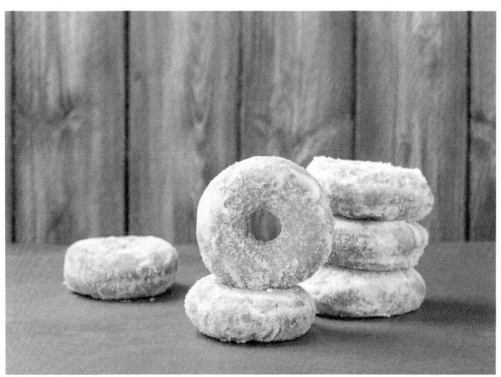

- **Preparation: 12 hours and 20 minutes**
- **Cooking time: 8 minutes**
- **Difficulty: Very easy**
- **Servings: 8**

INGREDIENTS
- 250g Flour
- 150g boiled Potatoes
- 1 Egg yolk
- 50g Butter
- 2 g fresh Brewer's yeast
- 1 pinch Fine salt
- 30g Sugar
- 25ml Oil
- Small amount of milk or water

PREPARATION
Prepare the dough at least 12 hours in advance so as to obtain perfect leavening.
You can proceed by kneading by hand, on a pastry board, or in the mixer.
Put the flour in the bowl of the mixer. In the centre, add the boiled potatoes (mashed). Add the egg yolk then the soft butter and the yeast dissolved in very little water or milk. Finally, add a pinch of salt and knead.
Knead it by hand on a pastry board to give it the shape of a loaf and put it to rise in a lightly floured bowl for 10 hours.
In the morning, turn the dough over onto the floured work surface, roll it out with a rolling pin and cut out the donuts with two cookie sizes of different diameters or a special mould.
Place each donut on a square of parchment paper and cover with a clean cloth.
Let it rise again for 2 hours until doubled.

COOKING SUGAR DONUTS IN AIR FRYER
Cut out the parchment paper following the shape of the donut.
Preheat the air fryer at 200°c for 3 minutes then place the donuts on the basket.
Sprinkle them with a few puffs of oil to cover them entirely.
Cook them for 2-3 minutes then turn them, removing the parchment paper, then sprinkle them again with a little oil and cook for another 2 minutes. After cooking, pass them in sugar.

POTATO BALLS

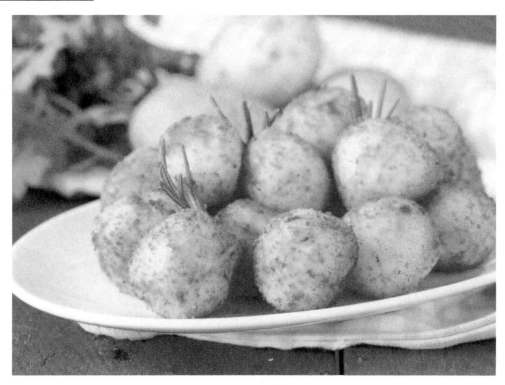

- **Preparation: 50 minutes**
- **Cooking time: 5 minutes**
- **Difficulty: Very easy**
- **Servings: 4**

INGREDIENTS
- 600g Potatoes
- 1 Egg
- 100g Breadcrumbs
- 60g Parmesan
- Salt
- Pepper
- Mint
- Oil

PREPARATION
Put the potatoes in a saucepan, add boiling water and coarse salt and place on high heat.
Cook them until tender: it will take about 15-20 minutes, depending on the size and variety. Cool them down for a few minutes, then remove the skin, place them in a mixing bowl and mash with a potato masher. Add the breadcrumbs, grated parmesan, egg, and mint (finely chopped). Season with salt and pepper and mix until you get well combined mixture. Let it rest for at least 20 minutes. Then make into small balls.

COOKING POTATO BALLS IN THE AIR FRYER
Preheat the fryer to 170°c, grease it with a drizzle of oil and the potato balls, frying them for 4-5 minutes.

PORCINI MUSHROOMS

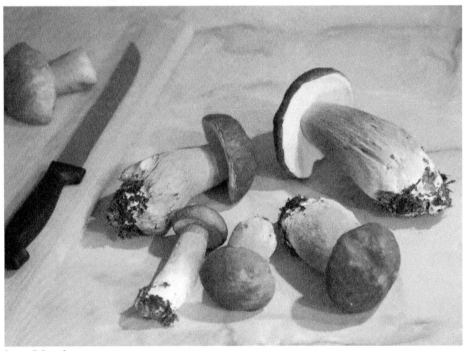

- **Preparation: 20 minutes**
- **Cooking time: 10 Minutes**
- **Difficulty: Easy**
- **Servings: 4**

INGREDIENTS
- 10 hats Porcini mushrooms
- 2 Eggs, beaten
- Flour
- Breadcrumbs
- 1 Lemon
- Salt
- Non-stick cooking spray

PREPARATION
Carefully clean the caps of the porcini mushrooms, lightly flour them, pass them quickly in the beaten eggs and then in the breadcrumbs, which must be very fine.

COOKING PORCINI MUSHROOMS IN THE AIR FRYER
Preheat the air fryer to 180°c, grease the fryer with a non-stick spray and fry the mushrooms for about 10 minutes. Serve with a squeeze of lime and a pinch of salt.

CAIPIRINHA CRAB CLAWS

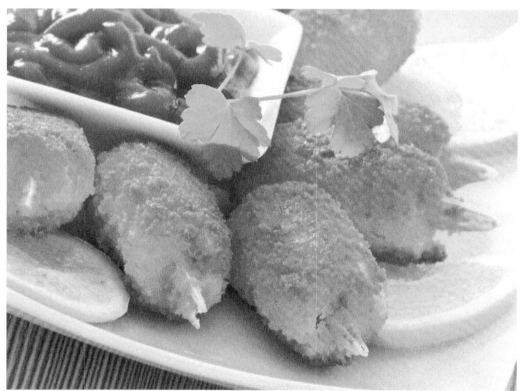

- **Preparation: 30 minutes**
- **Cooking time: 5 minutes**
- **Difficulty: Very easy**
- **Servings: 4**

INGREDIENTS
- 1 pack Crab claws (thawed)
- 1 piece Ginger
- 1 Lemon
- 2 Eggs
- 2 tablespoons Soy sauce

- Breadcrumbs
- Oil

PREPARATION

In a bowl, add the crab claws in a mixture of ginger, lemon juice, and soy. Beat the eggs and dip each claw into them. Finally pass them in the breadcrumbs.

COOKING CAIPIRINHA CRAB CLAWS IN AIR FRYER

Preheat the fryer to 170°c and grease it with a drizzle of oil.
Pour in the crab claws and fry them for about 5 minutes.

COURGETTE MUFFIN

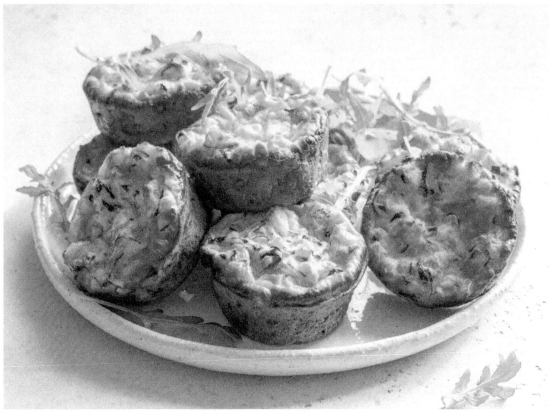

- **Cooking: 15 minutes**
- **Preparation: 10 minutes**
- **Difficulty: Very easy**
- **Servings: 12**

INGREDIENTS

- 200g Courgettes
- 20g Extra virgin olive oil
- 70g Butter
- 2 Eggs
- 100g Milk
- 250g Flour
- 100g grated Parmesan cheese
- ½ sachet Yeast
- Salt to taste

PREPARATION

Cut the courgettes into pieces. Sauté them in a pan for 2-3 minutes with the oil and butter. Blend the flour with the parmesan, eggs, milk, and a pinch of salt. Add the yeast and blend for a few more seconds. Finally, add the courgette. Add to the mixture. Pour the mixture into muffin cups filling them for ¾. Sprinkle the surface with grated parmesan cheese.

COOKING COURGETTE MUFFIN IN AIR FRYER

Cook for 15 minutes in an air fryer at 180°c.

TART OF COURGETTE

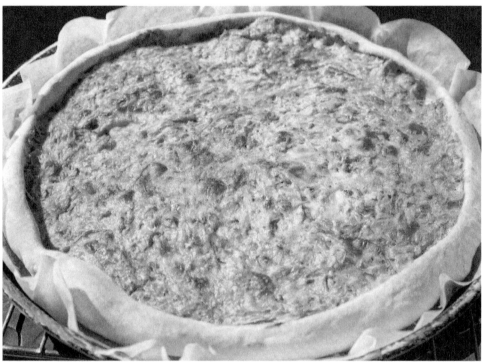

- **Preparation: 15 minutes**
- **Cooking: 25 minutes**
- **Difficulty: Medium**
- **Servings: 4**

INGREDIENTS
- 1 pack Puff pastry
- 600g Courgettes
- 2 Eggs (beaten)
- 2 Tomatoes
- ½ Onion
- 2 tablespoons Extra virgin olive oil
- 50g Parmesan
- Salt

PREPARATION

Chop and brown the onion, add the courgettes cut into slices, allow to flavour, then add the chopped tomatoes. Place in a pan and cook for 3-5 minutes. Remove from the heat and add the 2 beaten eggs and the parmesan. Roll out the puff pastry in a greased pan, up to the edges and arrange the mixture in it. Cover with the rest of the pastry.

COOKING TART OF COURGETTE IN THE FRYER
Preheat the fryer to 200°c, place the pan inside and cook for about 25 minutes.

FRENCH TOAST

- Preparation: 10 minutes
- Cooking time: 10 minutes
- Difficulty: Very easy
- Servings: 1

INGREDIENTS
- 1 Brioche bun
- 100g Cream cheese
- 2 Eggs
- 15ml Milk
- 30ml Cream
- 38g Sugar
- 3g Cinnamon
- 2ml Vanilla extract
- Non-stick cooking spray
- 20g chopped Pistachios, for garnish

PREPARATION
Wisk the eggs with the sugar and the cinnamon, add the milk, cream, and the vanilla. Dip each side of the toast into the and rest it on a grid or a flat tray.

COOKING FRENCH TOAST IN AIR FRYER
Turn on the air fryer and set the temperature to 180°c.
Place the toast in the preheated fryer and cook for 10 minutes.
Carefully remove the toast with a spatula when cooked. Serve with chopped pistachios and maple syrup.

DESSERTS

CAKE WITH WILD BERRIES

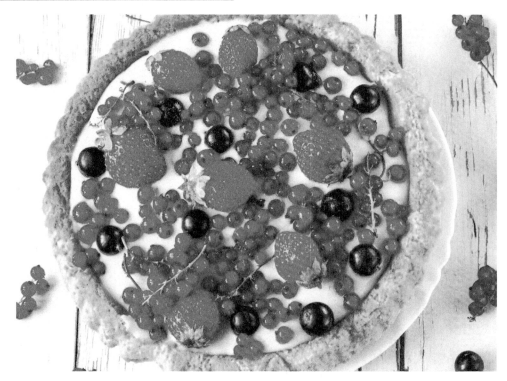

- **Preparation: 10 minutes**
- **Cooking time: 35 minutes**
- **Difficulty: Very easy**
- **Servings: 4**

INGREDIENTS
- 2 Eggs
- 100g Cane sugar
- 200g Buckwheat flour
- 50g Potato starch
- 100g Soy cream
- 120g Berries
- 10g Baking powder

PREPARATION
Whip the whole eggs with the sugar until a frothy mixture is obtained. Gradually add the buckwheat flour and the potato starch. Also add the baking powder. Set aside.
You can combine the berries with a spatula so as not to break them, leaving some to decorate on the surface.
Pour the rather thick mixture into a 22cm cake mould suitable for the basket of the air fryer.

COOKING CAKE WITH WILD BERRIES IN AIR FRYER
Place the mould on the basket and turn it on at 160°c, then cook for about 35 minutes. Allow to cool then top with berries.

CHOCOLATE MUFFIN

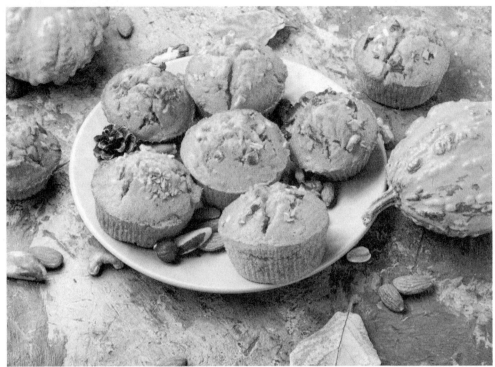

- **Preparation: 10 minutes**
- **Cooking time: 15 minutes**
- **Difficulty: Very easy**
- **Servings: 6**

INGREDIENTS
- 50g Granulated sugar
- 130ml Coconut or soy milk
- 60ml Coconut oil
- 5ml Vanilla extract
- 120g Flour
- 14g Cocoa powder
- 4g Baking powder
- 2g Baking soda
- A pinch of salt
- 80g Chocolate chips
- 25g Pistachio
- Non-stick cooking spray

PREPARATION
In a small bowl mix the sugar, with the coconut oil, vanilla and coconut milk.
In a separate bowl mix flour, baking powder, baking soda, salt and cocoa powder.
Combine both mixture together with the chocolate chips and pistachio until well incorporated and smooth. Once ready, place the mixture in the muffin paper cups.

COOKING CHOCOLATE MUFFINS IN AIR FRYER
Turn on the air fryer and set the temperature to 150°c.
Carefully place the muffin cups into the preheated fryer and cook for 15 minutes using the dessert option settings.
Remove the muffins when ready and let them cool for 10 minutes before serving.

BLUEBERRIES MUFFIN

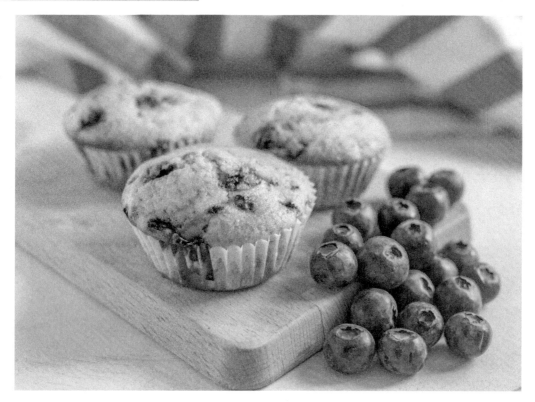

- **Preparation: 10 minutes**
- **Cooking time: 15 minutes**
- **Difficulty: Very easy**
- **Servings: 6**

INGREDIENTS
- 120g Flour
- 60g Sugar
- 4g Baking powder
- 2g Baking soda
- 100g Blueberries
- 1 egg
- 80ml Orange juice
- 60ml Vegetable oil
- 1 Orange (zest)
- Non-stick cooking spray
- Salt to taste

PREPARATION
Combine the eggs with the orange juice, zest and oil.
Mix together the flour, sugar, baking powder, baking soda, salt, and blueberries in a large bowl. Combine both mixture together until well incorporated and place it into the muffin moulds.

COOKING BLUEBERRY MUFFINS IN AIR FRYER
Turn on the air fryer and set the temperature to 160°c. Carefully place the muffin cups into the preheated fryer. Select the Desserts option, adjust the time to 15 minutes and let it cook.

AMARETTI WITH COCONUT

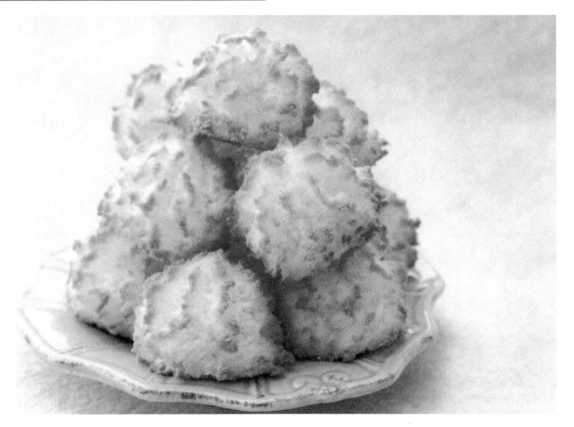

- **Preparation: 10 minutes**
- **Cooking time: 15 minutes**
- **Difficulty: Very easy**
- **Servings: 6**

INGREDIENTS
- 100g Milk
- 1 Egg white
- 2ml Almond extract
- 2ml Vanilla extract
- A pinch of salt
- 180g Unsweetened coconut (chopped)

PREPARATION
Mix the milk, egg white, almond extract, vanilla extract, and salt together in a bowl.
Add 160g of grated coconut and mix until well combined.
Shape into balls of about 40mm with your hands. On a separate plate, then add 20g of grated coconut.
Toss the amaretti in the grated coconut until covered.

COOKING AMARETTI WITH COCONUT IN AIR FRYER
Turn on the air fryer and set the temperature to 150°c.
Add the coconut amaretti to the preheated fryer. Select the Desserts option, adjust the time to 15 minutes and let it cook. Let the macaroons cool down for 10-15 minutes before serving.

LEMON CAKE

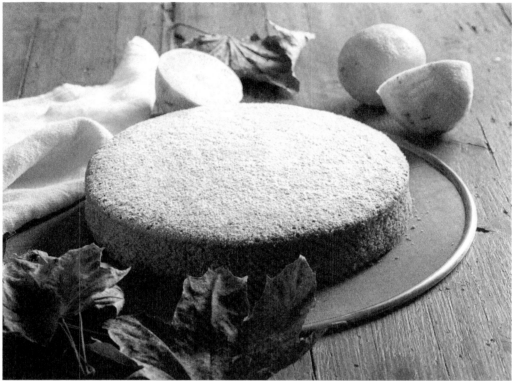

- **Preparation: 10 minutes**
- **Cooking time: 30 minutes**
- **Difficulty: Very easy**
- **Servings: 2**

INGREDIENTS
- 120g Flour
- 4g Baking powder
- A pinch of salt
- 80g Unsalted butter (softened)
- 130g Granulated sugar
- 1 Large egg
- 15g Fresh lemon juice
- 2 Lemons
- 50g Buttermilk

PREPARATION
Mix the flour, baking powder, and salt together in a bowl.

Mix the softened butter with a mixer for about 3 minutes until light and fluffy and then add the sugar and whip for an extra minute.

Stir the flour mixture into the butter, until completely incorporated. Add the egg, lemon juice, and lemon zest. Stir slowly until completely blended. Slowly pour in the milk and mix on medium speed. Pour the mixture into a mould of about 20 cm.

COOKING LEMON CAKE IN AIR FRYER
Turn on the air fryer and set the temperature to 160°c.

Place the cake in the preheated fryer. Cook for 30 minutes with the bread cooking settings.

CAPPUCCINO CAKE

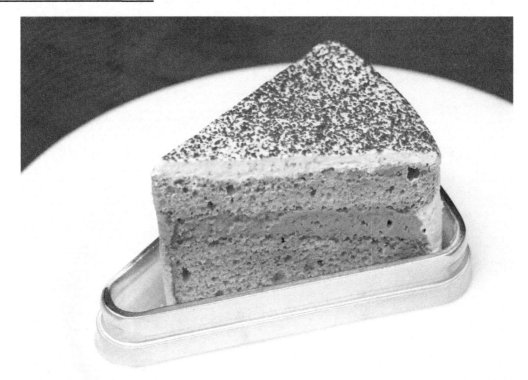

- **Preparation: 40 minutes**
- **Cooking time: 30 minutes**
- **Difficulty: Very easy**
- **Servings: 6**

INGREDIENTS
- 230g Flour
- 2 Eggs
- 140g Granulated sugar
- 40ml Milk
- 30ml Seed oil
- 60ml Coffee
- 100g Dark chocolate
- 1 sachet Baking powder

PREPARATION
Whip the whole eggs with the sugar using an electric whisk or in a mixer for at least 5 minutes at high speed until they are fluffy and foamy.
Add milk and oil slowly by lowering the speed of the electric whips. Finally, also add the lukewarm coffee.
Sift the flour with the baking powder and add the mix to the egg mixture, a little at a time and gently incorporating it. Chop the chocolate and incorporate it to the dough using a spatula. Leave some for the surface.
Pour the mixture into a 20cm mould lined with parchment paper and level it well. On the surface, add the remaining dark chocolate.

COOKING IN CAPPUCCINO CAKE AIR FRYER
Place the mould on the basket of the air fryer and cook for 20 minutes at 160°c then for 10 minutes at 180°c until the cooking is checked with a wooden toothpick.

CRUMBLED NUTELLA AND MASCARPONE

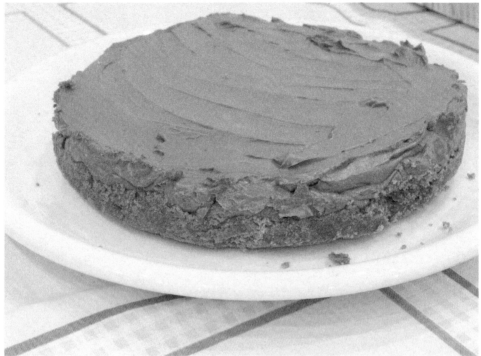

- **Preparation: 25 minutes**
- **Cooking: 25 minutes**
- **Difficulty: Very easy**
- **Servings: 4**

INGREDIENTS
For the Chocolate Shortbread
- 230g Flour
- 20g Bitter cocoa
- 100g Butter
- 1 Egg
- 2 teaspoons Baking powder
- 100g Granulated sugar

For the stuffing
- 250g Mascarpone
- 1 Egg yolk
- Nutella

PREPARATION
Prepare the shortcrust pastry, proceeding by hand or with a mixer.

Put the flour and cocoa on the work surface or in the bowl of the mixer.

Add the sugar, baking powder, and whole egg.

Finally, add the cold butter in chunks. Knead until you get a soft pastry.

Divide the dough into two equal parts and line a 20cm mould with parchment paper (if necessary).

Prepare the cream: mix the mascarpone with the yolk with a spatula, choose whether to sweeten it or not with the Nutella (I liked it with and without).

Crumble half the pastry into the mould both on the base and on the edges, compacting well and avoiding holes.

Then, add the mascarpone cream on the crumbled base and then the Nutella (if necessary, melted in a bain-marie or in the microwave).

COOKING CRUMBLED NUTELLA AND MASCARPONE IN AIR FRYER
Place the mould on the basket of the air fryer and cook at 170°c degrees for 15 minutes then at 190°c for another 10-15 minutes. You can also use the "cakes" mode if available for the same time, checking the cook after 25-30 minutes.

APPLE FRITTERS

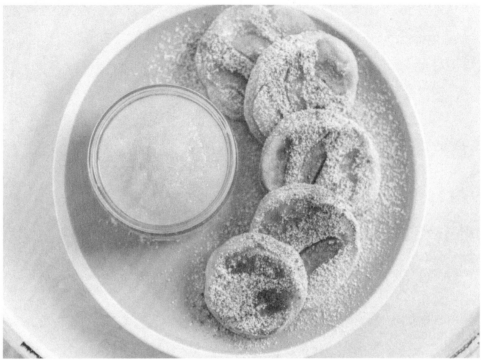

- **Preparation: 10 minutes**
- **Cooking time: 8 minutes**
- **Difficulty: Very easy**
- **Servings: 4**

INGREDIENTS
- 1 and a half cups Buckwheat flour
- 2 tablespoons Coconut sugar
- 2 teaspoons Baking powder
- ¼ teaspoon Vanilla extract
- 2 teaspoons Ground cinnamon
- 1 cup Almond milk
- 1 tablespoon Flaxseed
- 1 cup of sliced Apples
- 1 teaspoon Vegetable oil

PREPARATION
In a bowl, mix the flour with the sugar, baking powder, vanilla extract, and cinnamon.
Add the flaxseed, milk, and apple, and mix well until you get the pancake batter. Form pancakes with your hands about 7-8 cm in diameter and place them on a sheet of baking paper for the fryer.

COOKING APPLE FRITTERS IN AIR FRYER
Insert the pastry into the fryer and cook at 180°c for 7-8 minutes, turning them halfway through cooking.

CHOCOLATE COOKIES

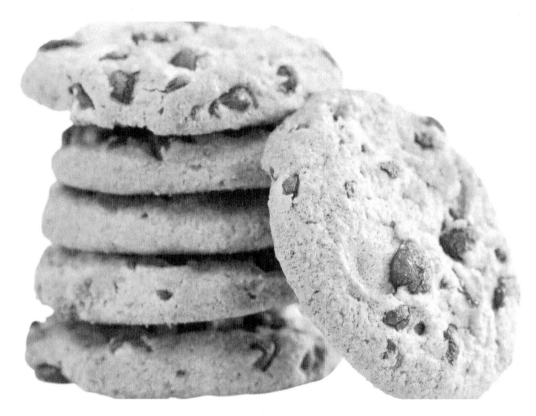

- **Preparation: 15 minutes**
- **Cooking time: 8 minutes**
- **Difficulty Very easy**
- **Servings: 5**

INGREDIENTS
- 300g Flour
- 2 Eggs
- 100g Granulated sugar
- 70ml Seed oil
- 1 teaspoon Baking powder
- 100g Chocolate chips

PREPARATION
Mix the flour with the eggs, oil, sugar, and yeast. Add the chocolate chips and form a loaf and form a firm dough. Lightly flour the work surface and work the dough, then cut into pieces, trying to give them the same weight, about 2 cm thick. Finally, place them on a pan that fits your air fryer.

COOKING CHOCOLATE COOKIES IN AIR FRYER
Place the pan on the basket with a sheet of parchment paper and cook at 160°c for 8 minutes flipping them halfway through

Printed in Great Britain
by Amazon

17207114R00045